Mediterranean Dash Diet Cookbook

90-Day Dash Diet Meal Plan For Beginners To Lose Weight And Lower Your Blood Pressure

#2020

By Mark Arizona

Table of Contents

Salad Recipes

Kale: A Versatile Superfood with Many Options

133. Peach Smoothie
134. Blueberry Smoothie
135. Blueberry Yogurt Smoothie
136. Blackberry, Blueberry, and Cherry Smoothie
137. Cherry and Banana Smoothie
138. Currents and Berries Smoothie with Yogurt
139. Pumpkin Spice Smoothie
140. Banana and Pumpkin Smoothie
141. Chocolate and Peanut Butter Smoothie
142. Chocolate and Banana Smoothie
143. Hazelnut and Chocolate Smoothie
144. Tahini and Honey Smoothie
145. Creamy Banana Smoothie
146. Cinnamon Banana Smoothie
147. Pistachio Smoothie
148. Banana and Pistachio Smoothie
149. Mocha Smoothie
150. Pumpkin and Banana Smoothie

Fresh Pressed Juices

151. Mango Carrot Juice
152. Kale and Apple Juice
153. Grapefruit Juice
154. Lemon and Apple Juice
155. Ginger Carrot Juice
156. Pineapple and Coconut Juice
157. Parsley, Beet and Carrot Juice
158. Turmeric, Apple and Lemon Juice
159. Watermelon and Mint Juice
160. Grape and Lime Juice
161. Pineapple and Coconut Juice
162. Turmeric, Ginger and Lemon Juice

Natural Flavor Infused Water

163. Cucumber Water
164. Citrus Water
165. Strawberries and Cucumber Water

on rare occasions?

Question: Should all salt be avoided, or is it permissible to enjoy a small amount every day?

Question: How much sugar is too much and when should it be avoided?

Question: How many eggs can be consumed daily?

Question: Are there any herbs or spices that should be avoided on the Dash diet?

Question: What is the difference between dark and milk chocolate? Does it matter which one I use in recipes?

Question: Is there enough protein in nuts and seeds for a vegan diet? Should I also include soy food options?

Question: Should portion control be a factor for more than just lean meats? Should I be limiting the amount of each food item and recipes I try and is there a guideline to follow?

Question: How do I avoid choosing the wrong foods when traveling or visiting another region or country where my regular meal options are not available?

Question: Are there limitations for older adults and the types of foods they can choose in the Dash diet?

Question: Is the Dash diet affordable?

Question: Is it important to be active and exercise with the Dash diet?

Question: How successful is the Dash diet?

CHAPTER 1: INTRODUCTION

What is the Dash Diet and How Can it
Improve Your Overall Health

The Dash diet was developed for the purpose of lowing blood pressure, increasing immunity and to promote weight loss. It stands for Dietary Approaches to Stop Hypertension and is strongly supported by medical professionals and dieticians as a safe, healthy way to live and eat well while maintaining normal blood pressure. It is a balanced diet that is recommended by the Kidney Foundation and the United States Department of Agriculture. The main goal of the diet is to focus on reducing meal portions and adding as many nutrients as possible, such as potassium, calcium, and magnesium, while significantly reducing sodium. Other characteristics of this diet include:

- Increasing the number of fresh fruits and vegetables
- Reducing red meats, skipping them completely
- Lean cuts of meat, such as poultry and seafood
- Low or non-fat dairy foods or plant-based substitutes
- Raw seeds and nuts
- Beans and sprouts
- Avoiding all (or most) processed and "junk" foods

In general, include as many wholes, natural food options as possible and increase the number of plant-based items in your diet for best results.

The Benefits of Adapting to the Dash Diet

The main goal of the Dash diet is reducing blood pressure and maintaining healthy levels. For many people who do not have high blood pressure, they may experience hypertension, which is an early sign that can lead to an increase in pressure, depending on your diet and lifestyle. Hypertension is often monitored to ensure that it does not increase, as this can lead to a higher risk of heart disease, heart attacks and impairment of the kidneys. It's a common condition in North America and is often linked to a poor diet and an inactive lifestyle, as main factors.

How is blood pressure measured? When you have your blood pressure measured, you'll notice two numbers. The first or top number is referred to as the systolic pressure. This indicates the pressure while your heart is pumping blood. The second or bottom number is diastolic pressure, which measures your heart when it's at rest. A normal or healthy blood pressure reading will show a higher number (systolic) between 120 and 140. The lower number should fall between 80-90. Low blood pressure refers to numbers that fall below 120 (systolic) and 80 (diastolic), while high blood pressure becomes a concern once the numbers reach over 140 (systolic) or over 90 (diastolic). Maintaining a healthy blood pressure level is crucial to staying healthy and avoiding serious medical conditions.

There are other benefits that may result from this way of eating, including weight loss, preventing type 2 diabetes, lowering cholesterol and increasing your body's metabolic function. If you lead an active lifestyle, the Dash diet will support your body with a significant amount of energy, including protein, calcium, vitamins, and minerals. Overall, the dietary requirements are easy to follow, and recipes are delicious, versatile and can be easily altered to meet your needs.

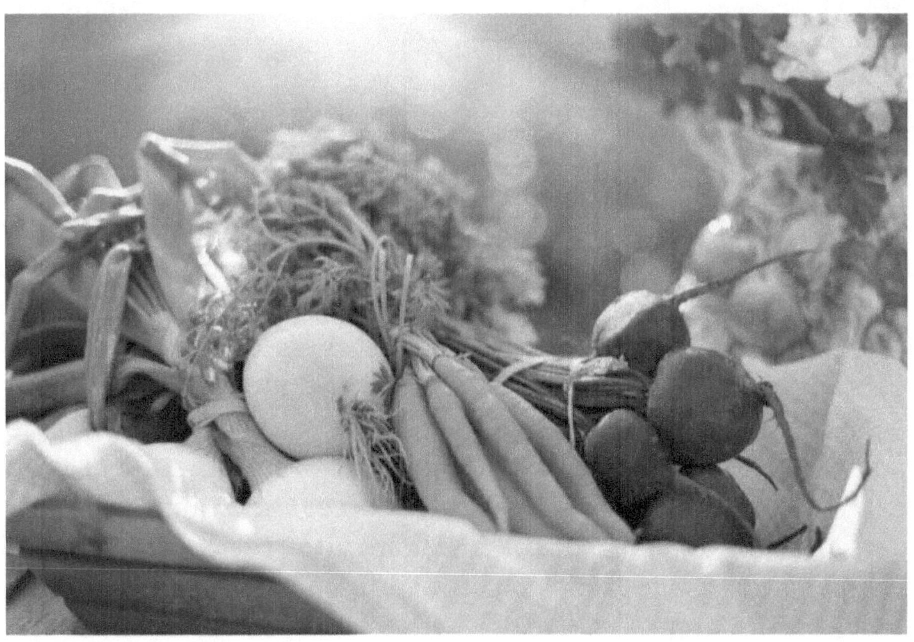

CHAPTER 2: FOODS TO INCLUDE IN THE DASH DIET

Foods that Promote Health

The first step to beginning the Dash diet is understanding the importance of key healthy foods high in nutrients and making them a part of your daily meals. If you already choose fresh produce and whole foods, you're on the right track. This diet focuses on getting the most out of natural food sources and skipping the processed snacks and meal options that are often too common in our weekly grocery shopping. The types of foods to focus on including the following:

- Fresh fruits, especially option high in antioxidants and vitamins. All fruits are a good source of fiber, which is vital for a healthy diet
- Select fresh vegetables at part of your grocery list, and choose dark, leafy greens to enhance the iron, calcium and protein sources, especially if you are vegan or limit your intake of animal protein.
- Skip processed foods and refined carbohydrates. If you choose a sweetener, consider organic honey or maple syrup, or choose a low carb sweetener. Low carb sweeteners, such as swerve, erythritol and monk fruit are excellent for minimizing the impact on glucose levels and play a major role in ketogenic diets and meal plans that significantly reduce carbohydrates.
- Focus on lean meats and seafood. Red meat, if consumed, should be chosen in its leanest form, and in smaller portions. Salmon, white fish, tuna and lean poultry are good choices for meat, while eggs and natural, low-fat dairy products are also a good choice, in

moderate amounts.

- Seeds and nuts, unsalted and unflavored, are good choices for highly nutritious snacks and food on the go

Foods that promote good health are more affordable than you may think!

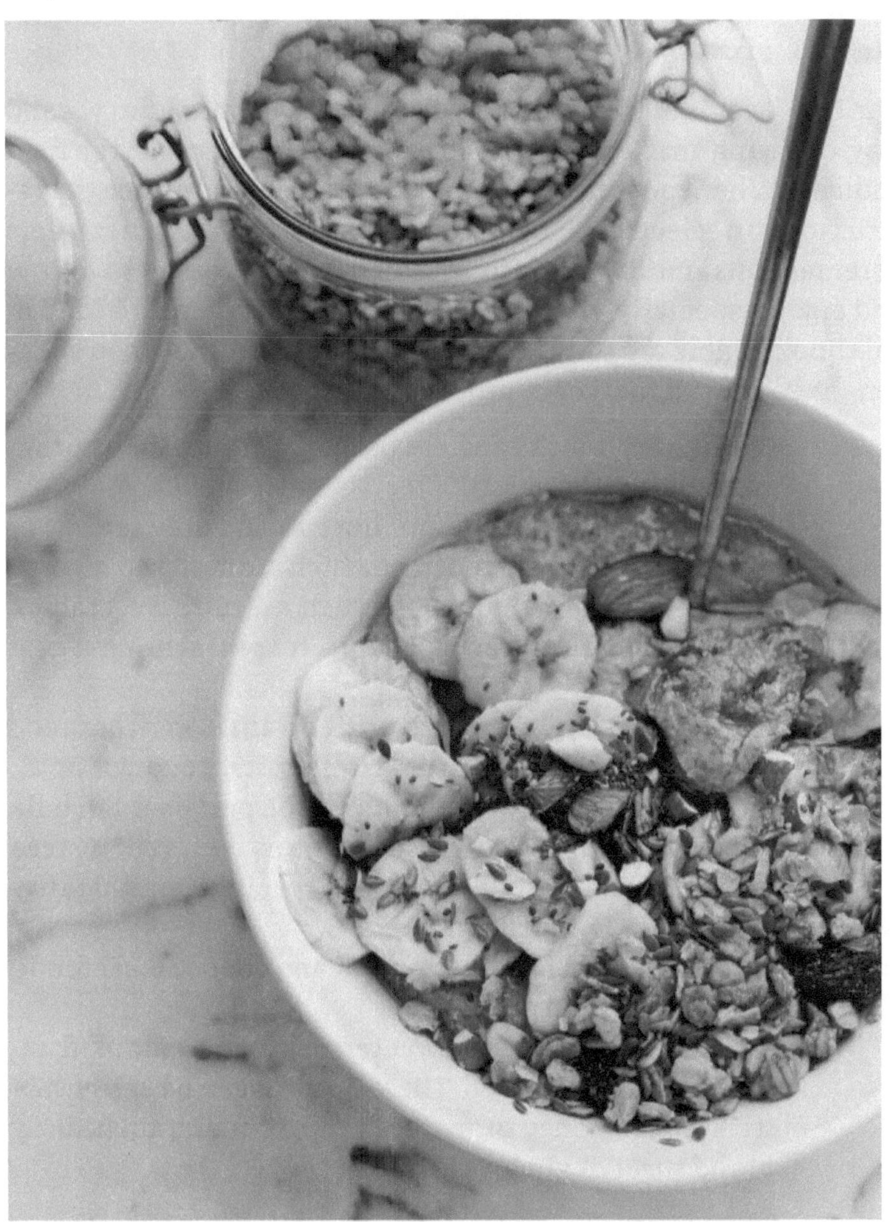

CHAPTER 3: HOW TO BEGIN THE DASH DIET

Choosing Foods and Ingredients for Simple, Healthy Recipes

The Dash Diet is more than just a diet; it's a healthier lifestyle and way of eating that ensures you get the most out of better food choices. When most people think of diets, they consider the restrictions on selection and portion control. The Dash diet offers a tremendous amount of options, which makes it easier to follow and enjoy, especially with the wide range of recipes provided in this book. There are some key items to keep in mind when shopping at your local market or grocery store:

- Avoid salty snacks and choose low sodium foods or ingredients without salt
- If you use salt, limit the amounts, or add only sea salt or pink Himalayan salt, both of which are easier to digest.
- Choose natural, whole foods such as fruits, vegetables, and grains. If fresh isn't available, frozen is the next best option
- Check a local bulk store to buy certain items that tend to be costly, such as macadamia nuts, coconut or almond flour. Many ingredients can be purchased in bulk in the exact or approximate amount required, instead of buying one full box or bag of a specific item that may only be used in small amounts.
- Visit your local farmers' market and choose local foods, baked goods and produce
- Try different low carb sweeteners, such as monk fruit, swerve and erythritol. These options can be easily substituted for honey or maple syrup, to maintain healthy blood sugar or glucose levels.

Creating a Useful Shopping List

It may seem more challenging than you think, but choosing the right foods for your lifestyle can easily when you consider the types of fresh and frozen foods available. To build your shopping list, compare the items you currently select the types of foods that are suitable for a Dash diet plan, then consider the alternatives, if they are necessary. For example, if you choose 5-6 apples in a bag as part of your weekly shopping routine, this is already Dash diet-friendly and doesn't require any further changes. On the other hand, choosing sugary fruit snacks in the candy aisle is an example of an item that should be switched with fresh fruit or another wholesome food snack, such as almonds or peanuts.

The following examples or "starter recipes" can be helpful in providing a solution to what you may currently be buying versus better options:

1. Fresh almonds and sun-dried fruits
    - This is a good replacement for sugary fruit snacks or candies that may indicate natural flavors, only to include many unnatural ingredients as well

2. Sesame seeds with pink Himalayan salt or chili pepper
    - This is a good alternative to pretzels and other salty snacks that are high in sodium and additives.

3. Fresh peaches and pineapples with (or without)
a light drizzle of natural or low carb syrup.
    - Skip canned fruits completely for fresh options, and make them a part of your daily shopping list. Choosing fresh over canned is one of the most important changes you'll make in following this diet. While many people are accustomed to the sweet, dessert-like quality of canned fruit cocktails, peaches or pears, for example, they may not realize how high the sugar content is.

4. Plain yogurts and cream cheese products topped

with fresh fruits, nuts, and other toppings

- Avoid all flavored and sweetened items, including fruit-bottom yogurts, cream cheese, and other dairy products. Keep everything plain and if required, low-fat, to keep within your dietary guidelines. Choose natural options for flavor and focus on tailoring those choices to suit your desired tastes. For example, choosing your own custom selection of fruits, such as kiwi, oranges, and grapes, may seem less common than packaged, flavored products, though your advantages are: the flavors are chosen by you and they do not come with the added hidden sugars and additives.

5. Marinate your own meats and soy-based foods
(tofu and low sodium soy sauce)

- Avoid added sodium, nitrates and sugars by choosing to marinate your own foods. The only drawback is taking a bit more time than you may expect, though this can be easily settled into your schedule and done with ease over time. Marinating your own foods gives you the option of selecting the exact flavor combination you want while learning to understand what creates the types of tastes you're looking for. This can include sweet or sour, sweet and spicy, tangy, spicy and tart, etc.

CHAPTER 4: RECIPES FOR SOUPS, SALADS AND LIGHT MEALS TO START

Soups and Broths

An easy way to start the Dash diet is to start with a simple broth or soup. Add one or two cups to your diet each week and try a few different options to get an idea of which flavors you prefer. Broths are generally easy to prepare and involve boiling the carcass of leftover roast beef, chicken or turkey. The process requires some time management, as creating a high-quality bone broth requires cooking the bones anywhere between 20-24 hours.

1. Chicken Bone Broth

To prepare for a chicken broth, it's an advantage if you have a left-over roast chicken, where all the bones can be removed, dried and set aside. A local butcher or the meat section in a grocery store can provide bones as well if you want to skip the roast dinner.

- Bones from the carcass of one chicken
- 6-8 cups of water (or enough to cover the bones in a large cooking pot)
- Sea salt or pink Himalayan salt (in small amounts, or a low-sodium alternative)

Place all the chicken bones from one carcass into a large cooking pot and cover with water. Bring to a boil on medium-high heat and maintain the boil for at least ten minutes. Add salt as desired and reduce heat to medium or medium-low and continue to cook for another hour. Reduce heat further to cook on low. If you prepare this broth at night, leave the pot on low heat, or turn it off completely and continue to cook, covered, while supervised. Allow the bones to remain in the water for up to 24 hours. Taste test every few hours and add more salt if desired.

Once the broth is done, pour the liquid into another large or medium cooking pot while draining from the bones. Add any other spices (a little salt or an alternative), then transfer to a sealed container and refrigerate. Keep in the refrigerator for up to one week, or freeze longer, up to two months.

Note: for this and other broth recipes, limit the amount of salt used or use an alternative to salt that is low in sodium. If you choose salt, select sea salt or the pink Himalayan salt as they are better absorbed by your body.

2. Turkey Bone Broth

Turkey bone broth is a great option after a festive dinner, as is can provide a lot of nutrients as a light second meal, as a soup base or a simple broth on its own. Preparing a turkey broth is the same process as chicken, including the time frame. To enhance the flavor of this broth, add sage, poultry spices, and thyme.

3. Beef Bone Broth

Beef bone broth contains a few nutrients not included in poultry broths: iron and higher levels of protein. If you need a boost in both nutrients, beef is a good option and can provide a healthy dose of both in a small portion. To prepare this broth, use the bones of a leftover roast dinner or a local butcher. Bring them to a boil in a large pot, covered in water, and simmer for 22-24 hours. No salt or spices are necessary, though if you choose to add a little flavor, black pepper or dried garlic are good options. Avoid salt or use a limited amount.

4. Vegetable Broth

If you follow a vegan or plant-based diet, this is an excellent alternative to meat-based bone broths. Creating a vegetable broth can include a lot of ingredients already in your refrigerator, as well as any discarded vegetable peelings, skins and stems removed and often discarded in an organic bin or compost. Consider some of the following options to include:

- Onion skins and peels
- Garlic stems, leftover cloves, and skins
- Carrot and parsnip peels
- Celery stems
- Bell pepper seeds, stems and leftover slices
- Dried herbs such as sage, basil, parsley
- Cabbage leaves and stems

In a large cooking pot, add all the ingredients listed above, including other peels, skins or sliced vegetables and herbs preferred. Cover with 6-8 cups of water and cover. Bring to a boil and allow the boiling to continue for approximately 15 minutes. Reduce heat to low-medium and cook for one hour, reducing the heat to low and cooking for another 22-24 hours. Stir every 1-2 hours and add any spices as desired, avoiding salt and/or sodium-based spices. Taste test every 2-4 hours and add more spices to enhance the flavor. After 24 hours, remove from heat and drain the broth into a sturdy resealable container and refrigerate or freeze.

Broth can be divided into smaller portions to freeze for a longer time. It's a great option to enjoy on its own or use it as a soup base to build your own creations or for other recipes.

5. Miso Soup

A popular soup in Asian cuisine, and often served in sushi restaurants as aside. Miso is a fermented soybean and its available in three varieties: Shiro miso (white paste, mild in flavor), Shinshu miso (yellow paste, mild to moderate in flavor) and Aka miso (red paste; strong, pungent in flavor).

Miso soup is prepared by combining boiling water with miso paste, which is available in most grocery stores. You may find more options in natural food stores and Asian grocers. Soup kits may also be available, providing small single-serving sized miso cups for a quick boost in between meals. Miso is full of nutrients, including B12, calcium, protein, iron, and fiber. It's a superfood that prevents cancer, strengthens the immune system and improves blood pressure and heart health. While miso naturally contains salt, it's just enough to give your body the required amount of sodium without any negative effects. In fact, miso is perfectly "salted" or seasoned on its own and is a great addition to many sauces, marinades, and soup bases.

Preparing miso soup is quick and simple, unlike making bone broth or vegetable stock from scratch:

- 2-3 cups water
- 3-4 teaspoons miso paste (Shiro or Shinshu)

If you prefer making miso soup from the pre-portioned kits, follow the instructions on the package. For miso paste, which is often available in a jar or carton, bring 2-3 cups of water to a boil in a medium saucepan and add the miso paste. Reduce heat to medium and stir steadily to ensure the miso fully dissolves and mixes evenly into the water. Serve in small bowls or in a cup. Miso soup can also be stored in the refrigerator for several days, though since it's quick to prepare, it's best to make the soup before consuming it.

Building Your Soup

Are you looking to add more to your broth and make it a more filling meal? There are plenty of heart-healthy options to consider, from simple variations to more complex layers of taste and spices. One or two ingredients can make an impact in a simple broth while experimenting with herbs and spices to add savory or pungent taste to a mild soup.

6. Egg Drop Soup

If you are looking for something a little more substantial than a broth, this is a tasty option, packed with protein and healthy fats. One egg is all that's needed for a single serving soup packed with protein, calcium and omega 3 and 6 fatty acids.

- 2 cups of broth (chicken or turkey)
- 1 egg (beaten, in a small bowl)

- ½ cup of cooked chicken or turkey (leftover from a roast)
- 1 sliced carrot
- 1 sliced celery stalk
- Black pepper

In a medium cooking pot, heat the broth and add the egg. Stir the egg so that it is separated and mixes into the soup. Add the cooked turkey or chicken, followed by the carrot, celery and sprinkle with black pepper. Reduce heat to low and stir for another 5 minutes before serving.

7. Traditional Miso Soup

Miso soup is an excellent base for many ingredients and flavoring. This recipe follows the most popular miso soup version, which is often served alongside sushi or sashimi dishes.

- 2-3 cups of prepared miso soup (Shiro miso)
- ½ cup of dried seaweed
- ¼ cup of sliced green onions
- ½ cup of soft tofu, sliced into small cubes

When preparing the miso soup, add the seaweed to the water and boil first, before adding the miso paste. Alternatively, add the seaweed into the miso soup after the paste has fully dissolved, then cook for at least 10-15 minutes until soft. Add the tofu and stir for another 5 minutes, then add the green onions, remove from heat and pour into cups or bowls to serve.

8. Mushroom Miso Soup

Mushrooms are an excellent ingredient for miso. They cook quickly and add a pleasant flavor, and contain fiber, minerals, and vitamins. Small, white mushrooms sliced thinly can be added to the miso broth and cooked for no more than 10 minutes before serving. Other varieties of mushrooms to consider include shiitake (large, dark grey in color) and Enokitake (long, thin stems resembling bean sprouts).

- 2-3 cups of prepared miso soup (Shiro or Shinshu miso)
- ½ cup thinly sliced white or shiitake mushrooms (or enokitake mushrooms, not sliced)
- Black pepper (optional)

Add the mushrooms to a cooking pot of prepared miso soup and cook on medium heat for 10-15 minutes, or until the mushrooms are soft. Add a teaspoon of black pepper, if desired, and serve.

9. Cabbage and Carrot Miso Soup

This is a simple soup created from a miso base, though it can be prepared with chicken or vegetable broth as well.

- 2 cups of prepared miso soup (Shiro miso)
- ¼ cup of shredded carrots
- ½ cup of shredded or thinly sliced cabbage leaves

After preparing the miso soup base, add the shredded carrots and cabbage, then reduce heat to medium and continue to stew until softened, about 15 minutes. Serve in a bowl or cup.

10. Chili Pepper Miso Soup

Spicy miso is a great addition as a side to baked salmon or a meal-sized salad. To enhance the soup base, add ½ cup of beef or chicken broth, or use less water to intensify the miso flavor. You may want to use Shinshu or Aka miso or combine a little of each to create a stronger taste or use the Shiro on its own.

- 2-3 cups of water
- 2-3 teaspoons miso paste (or a combination of two miso paste options)
- ½ cups of chicken or beef broth (optional)
- 3 tablespoons thinly sliced or dried and crumbled chili peppers
- ¼ cups of sliced green onions

Bring the 2-3 cups of water to a boil and add the miso paste, chili pepper and broth (optional). Lower the heat to medium and cook for another 15 minutes. Add the green onions and serve.

11. Miso Soup with Ramen Noodles

This recipe creates a fuller meal with whole-grain ramen noodles. Only a handful are needed to add for texture and sustenance. Other ingredients are optional: mushrooms, green onion, peppers, seaweed, and other vegetables you may have left in your refrigerator.

- 3 cups of prepared miso soup (Shiro or Shinshu miso)
- 1 handful of ramen noodles
- ¼ cup of green onions
- ¼ cup of sliced mushrooms
- Pinch of black pepper

Prepare three cups of miso soup and add the noodles. Bring to a boil until the ramen is cooked, then reduce heat and add all the remaining ingredients (except the green onions) and cook for 15 minutes on medium. Remove from heat and serve topped with green onions.

Hearty Soups

The earlier recipes in this chapter focus on creating a broth, either from meat bones, vegetables or miso paste, and adding simple ingredients. The following recipes build upon the soup base options, by combining simple flavors and ingredients that provide easy meal solutions.

12. Chicken Noodle Soup

- 2-3 cups of chicken broth
- 1 cup of cooked chicken breast, cut into one-inch pieces
- I chopped carrot
- ½ cup of peas (fresh or frozen)
- ½ cup of uncooked noodles

Heat the broth in a medium or large cooking pot with one additional cup of water and add the noodles. Bring to a boil, then reduce to medium to cook until tender. Add in the chicken and vegetables. Add seasonings, such as black pepper and turmeric, if desired, and serve.

13. Beef Barley Soup
- 2-3 cups of beef, chicken or vegetable broth
- 1 cup of uncooked barley
- 1 cup of cooked roast beef
- 2 celery stalks, chopped into small half-inch pieces
- I carrot, chopped
- I small onion, chopped finely
- 2 teaspoons dried parsley
- 1 teaspoon of black pepper

Heat the broth on medium and add an extra cup of water, if needed. Combine the barley and beef cubes and cook until tender. Add in the remaining ingredients, including the spices and cook for 30 minutes on medium.

14. Spinach and Broccoli Soup
- 1 cup of fresh spinach leaves
- 1 cup of broccoli florets, chopped into one-inch pieces
- 2 cups of chicken or vegetable broth
- 1 teaspoon miso paste
- ½ cup of sliced button mushrooms
- 1 onion, sliced finely
- 1 teaspoon of black pepper

In a large cooking pot, add the broth and spices, heating for 10 minutes on medium. Add the remaining ingredients and cook for 20 minutes, then serve.

15. Kidney Bean Stew
- 1 large can of kidney beans
- ½ cup of barley
- 3 cups of vegetable or beef broth
- 1 cup tomato juice
- Dash of black pepper
- 2 cloves of garlic, crushed
- 2 carrots sliced into small pieces

- 1 stalk of celery sliced

Kidney beans offer a significant source of fiber and protein. Barley and vegetables are added for more nutrients. This stew works best with canned beans, as they take less time to cook. To prepare this meal, add 3 cups of beef or vegetable broth in a large cooking pot and heat on medium. Add the beans, barley, garlic, carrots, and celery and cook for 30-40 minutes or until tender. Add the black pepper and serve.

16. Butternut Squash Soup
    - 3 cups of vegetable broth
    - 1 large or medium butternut squash (if not available, any variety of squash can be used for this recipe)
    - 2 potatoes
    - 1 teaspoon of black pepper
    - 2-3 tablespoons of olive oil
    - 1 carrot, chopped into small pieces
    - 1 teaspoon of thyme
    - 1 teaspoon of nutmeg (optional)
    - 1 tablespoon of butter
    - 2 stalks of celery, cut into small pieces
    - 1 small onion, diced

To prepare the squash for this soup, preheat the oven to 350 degrees. Prepare a baking sheet with parchment paper and bake the whole squash (with fork holes poked 2-3 times) for 30 minutes. Remove from the oven and slice in half. Remove the seeds and bake for another 10-15 minutes, until all flesh is soft, then scoop into a medium bowl and set aside.

In a large cooking pot, add the three cups of vegetable broth and bring to a boil. Add in the squash, potatoes (peeled and sliced into small, one-inch pieces), onion, celery, and carrots. Continue to cook and reduce the heat to medium for another 30 minutes, adding in the thyme, pepper, and nutmeg, then continue until potatoes are soft. Reduce heat to a low setting and remove the cooking pot. In small batches, pour the soup into a food processor or blender and pulse until smooth. Once all soup is blended, return to the cooking pot and return to medium heat. Add any additional seasonings, then serve.

17. Ginger Carrot Soup
- 2 onions, chopped
- 3-4 carrots, sliced into one-inch pieces
- ½ cup of sour cream
- 3 tablespoons of ground, fresh ginger
- 5-6 cups of chicken or vegetable broth
- 1 cup of whipping cream
- 2 teaspoons of butter
- Parsley or cilantro, for garnish

In a large cooking pot, bring the vegetable or chicken broth to a boil and add in the ginger, carrots, and onions. Cook until all ingredients are soft. As an alternative, use a skillet to fry the onions in 1-2 teaspoons of olive oil or butter, then add to the soup, along with the carrots and ginger. Reduce heat and remove the cooking pot and blend the soup in batches until smooth. Return the soup to the stove and heat on medium, stirring in the whipping cream and adding black pepper, if desired. Serve topped with sour cream and parsley or cilantro.

18. Sweet Potato Stew
- 2 large sweet potatoes, peeled and sliced
- 3 cups of chicken or vegetable broth
- 2 teaspoons of turmeric
- 1 teaspoon of black pepper
- 1 onion, diced
- 1 teaspoon of basil

Heat three cups of chicken or vegetable broth and add the potatoes and onions. Cook for 35-40 minutes, or until tender, then add the turmeric, basil, and black pepper. Remove from heat and pour the soup into the blender in batches, mixing until smooth. Return to the stove and heat, adding more seasoning and cooking for 5-10 minutes, then serve.

19. Potato and Leek Stew
- 3-4 medium or large potatoes, peeled and sliced
- 3 cups of chicken or vegetable broth
- 1 bunch of leeks, washed and sliced into one or two-inch pieces
- 1 teaspoon of black pepper
- 1 small onion, peeled and diced
- 1 teaspoon of turmeric
- ¼ cup of bacon bits (optional – may be real bacon or a vegetarian version)

Bring three cups of vegetable or chicken broth to a boil in a large cooking pot with the potatoes and onions. Cook until tender, and reduce heat, adding the black pepper and turmeric. Remove from heat and transfer to a blender in batches, mixing until smooth, then return to medium heat and add in the leeks, cooking for 10-15 minutes until tender. Stir in the bacon bits and serve.

20. Cream of Broccoli Soup
- 1 broccoli, chopped into small florets, including part of the stem (or this may be removed)
- 3 cups of chicken or vegetable broth
- 2 teaspoons of black pepper
- 1 onion, peeled and chopped
- 3 tablespoons of flour
- 2 cups of milk
- 2 stalks of celery, chopped
- 2 tablespoons of butter

In a skillet, heat two tablespoons of butter and add in the onion, celery, and broccoli. Cook for 10-12 minutes, then remove and add to a large cooking pot with 3 cups of broth. Bring to a boil on medium heat and cook for 20 minutes, then remove and blend in batches until smooth. Return to the cooking pot and cook for another 10 minutes on medium. In a skillet, add 1 teaspoon of butter, with the flour and milk and cook on low for 10 minutes. Pour into the soup and cook for another 10-15 minutes, then serve.

21. Broccoli Cheese Soup

This recipe follows the previous cream of broccoli ingredients and cooking instructions, plus adding 1 cup of shredded cheese on the skillet with the milk and flour, then pour into the soup and cook until all cheese is melted and mixed into the soup before serving. Add more cheese if necessary. Cheddar is recommended, though mozzarella is another option.

22. Curried Cauliflower Soup

- 1 roasted head of cauliflower, chopped into small florets
- 4 cups of vegetable or chicken broth
- 3 tablespoons of curry powder
- 1 teaspoon of turmeric
- 1 onion, peeled and diced
- 3 cloves of garlic, crushed
- 1 can of coconut milk

To prepare the cauliflower, preheat the oven to 350 degrees and place it on a baking tray. Bake for 30 minutes or until golden, then remove and chop into smaller pieces, then set aside. In a large cooking pot, add the broth, curry powder and coconut milk and bring to a boil on medium heat. Slice the cauliflower into smaller pieces and add to the pot with the garlic and onion. Continue cooking until all vegetables are tender, then transfer to a food processor and blend in batches. Return to the cooking pot and heat, then serve.

23-32. Light meals (3-4 ingredients combined in each recipe)

Lunch and dinner can be simplified with these quick recipes. These dishes can be prepared by combining several ingredients onto a platter or arranged in a resealable container for a portable lunch or snack option. The following "mini" recipes are heart-healthy and low in sodium.

23. Two hard-boiled eggs, 6-8 slices of cucumber and 4 cubes of low sodium cheddar cheese

24. Two slices of smoked salmon wrapped in low-fat cream cheese and capers

25. One large lettuce leaf wrap with chickpeas, sliced onion, and lemon juice

26. Light cream cheese and cucumber wrapped in lettuce leaves

27. Black olives, 4-6 cubes of low sodium mozzarella cheese and one cup of sliced carrots

28. One Sliced pomegranate into quarters, 4-5 cubes of feta cheese and one small apple

29. Sliced celery and carrots, both lengthwise, with a small cup of hummus

30. ½ cup of raw almonds, 1 cup of dried berries and apricots

31. ½ cup of cashews, 1 cup of dried cherries and ¼ cup of dried sliced coconut

32. 1 cup of unsalted peanuts, ½ cup of dried prunes and blueberries

Portable lunches and snacks are easy to prepare and go a long way to providing nutrients in between meals. They can help curb any cravings for salty or sugary snacks.

Salad Recipes

33. Tuna Salad
    - 1 can of tuna drained
    - 1 teaspoon of black pepper
    - 2 tablespoons of mayonnaise
    - 1 teaspoon of dried dill (optional)

- 2 teaspoons thinly sliced onion

Combine all ingredients into a small bowl. Serve on toast as an open-faced sandwich or in a grilled wrap

34. Spicy Tuna Salad

Following the ingredients listed in the above recipe, add 2 teaspoons of cayenne pepper and a dash of chili powder. Serve on bread.

35. Tuna and Cucumber Salad

- 1 cucumber, sliced into 1/2 -inch pieces
- 2 cans of tuna, drained
- 3 tablespoons of mayonnaise
- 1 stalk of celery, chopped into ½ inch pieces
- 1-2 teaspoons of black pepper

Combine all ingredients in a medium bowl and serve as a side or a snack.

36. Spicy Cucumber and Tuna Salad

Combine the ingredients in the above recipe and add one sliced jalapeno pepper and two crushed chili peppers.

37. Egg Salad

- 2 hard-boiled eggs
- 2 teaspoons of mayonnaise
- 1 teaspoon of dried dill
- 1 teaspoon of paprika

Mash three boiled eggs in a medium bowl and add in the mayonnaise, dill, and paprika. Serve on bread or as a side with salad.

38. Spinach and Egg Salad

- 1 cup of cooked spinach
- 3 hard-boiled eggs
- 2 teaspoons of mayonnaise
- 1 teaspoon of paprika
- 1 teaspoon of black pepper

Mash the eggs and add the spinach, then mayonnaise until evenly mixed. Add the paprika and black pepper, then serve. Make sure the cooked spinach is completely drained before adding to this recipe.

39. Salmon Salad
- 1 can of drained salmon
- 1 teaspoon of black pepper
- 1 teaspoon of sliced onion
- 2 teaspoons of mayonnaise

Drain and empty the salmon into a small bowl and mash until all the bones or cartilage are crushed or removed. Add the mayonnaise, onion and black pepper. Serve on rye bread.

40. Spicy Salmon Salad

Combine the ingredients in the above recipe and add 2 teaspoons of chili powder.

41. Coleslaw
- 2 cups of shredded carrots
- 1 ½ cups of shredded cabbage
- ½ cup of mayonnaise
- 1 teaspoon of vinegar
- 2 teaspoons of lemon juice
- 1 teaspoon of black pepper

Combine the mayonnaise, lemon juice, vinegar and black pepper in a small bowl and set aside. In a medium bowl, mix the shredded cabbage and carrots. Pour in the dressing and mix evenly. Sprinkle with fresh black pepper and serve

42. Coleslaw with dried berries

Combine the ingredients in the above recipe and top with ½ cup of dried blueberries or raisins.

43. Coleslaw Topped with Roasted Almonds

Prepare the coleslaw and heat a small skillet on low to medium heat. Toss ½ cup of sliced almonds and dry roast for 2-3 minutes or until slightly browned. Cool briefly and top the coleslaw

44. Simple Vinaigrette Salad Dressing Recipe

Creating a salad dressing that is healthy and budget-friendly only requires a few base ingredients plus the flavors of your choosing. Rosemary, mint, fruit extracts and juices, among many other options. It's an easy way to add zest to your salad without investing in high sugar or sodium-heavy dressings and sauces, which are also expensive!

Step 1:　　　　　Choose an oil to start your dressing. Olive oil, coconut or avocado oil are the best options

Step 2:　　　Vinegar is the next ingredient. Choose a rice or apple vinegar, either plain or something with a distinct flavor

Step 3:　　　Select your flavors. Garlic is great for adding a dose of nature's antibiotic. Natural fruit juice is great for antioxidants, vitamin C and A and a hint of sweetness. Maple syrup, mustard, chili pepper, and other unique tastes and combinations can be mixed into any custom form of vinaigrette you desire. For the Dash diet, avoid using salt or refined sugars, and choose from whole food sources, such as freshly squeezed fruit juices, dried herbs, and spices.

The following salad recipes are suitable for many vinaigrette options, with each recipe providing a recommended flavor to add to an oil and vinegar combination.

45. Arugula, Parmesan and Roasted Pear Salad
- 1 bunch of fresh arugula leaves
- ¼ cups of parmesan cheese shavings
- 1 pear, cut into quarters (oven roasted)
- ½ cup of crushed pecans

Wash and chop the arugula leaves and toss them into a bowl. Preheat the oven to 350 degrees to roast the pear. Slice the pear in half and core, then roast for 10-15 minutes or until tender. Cut into smaller pieces and add to the arugula. Toss in the parmesan and pecans, and serve with a simple vinaigrette (olive oil, apple cider vinegar, and blueberry juice are recommended).

46. Spinach and Blueberry Salad
- 1 bunch of fresh spinach leaves
- ½ cups of blueberry
- ¼ cup sliced almonds
- ¼ cup of shredded carrots
- ¼ cups of crumbled feta cheese (low sodium)

Wash and rinse spinach leaves, then add them to a large bowl with shredded carrot and fresh blueberries. Mix well, and top with sliced almonds and crumbled feta cheese. Serve with a vinaigrette flavored with fruit juice, such as raspberries or blueberries.

47. Walnut and Sprout Salad
- 2 cups of alfalfa or sesame seed sprouts
- ½ cups of crushed walnuts
- ½ cups of shredded carrots
- ½ cups of parsley, finely sliced

Wash and rinse the sprouts, adding into a large bowl. Toss in the shredded carrots and parsley, then blend and top with walnuts. Serve with a vinaigrette flavored with citrus juice (orange flavor suggested).

48. Chickpea Salad
- 1 can of chickpeas, drained and rinsed
- 1 cup of onion, peeled and diced
- 1 teaspoon of black pepper
- ½ cucumber, sliced into small, ½ inch pieces
- ½ cup of cherry tomatoes, sliced in half
- ½ green pepper sliced into ½ inch pieces
- 2 tablespoons dried parsley

Rinse a can of chickpeas and add to a medium bowl. Add the onions, green peppers, tomatoes and cucumber, and mix. Add in the parsley, black pepper and 2 teaspoons of vinegar and olive oil.

Combine thoroughly and serve.

49. Spicy Moong Bean Sprout Salad
- 1 large tomato, sliced into small cubes
- 1-2 small chilis, crushed with seeds
- 1 small onion, peeled and diced
- 1 teaspoon of lemon or lime juice
- 1 teaspoon of black pepper
- 1 teaspoon of chili powder

Steam the moong beans in a small or medium cooking pot until tender, then drain and add to a large bowl with all other ingredients. Mix well and serve. Top with coriander and lemon juice.

50. Apple and Kale Salad
- 1 bunch of kale, sliced with stems removed
- 1 crispy apple (Honeycrisp is recommended)
- 2 tablespoons freshly squeezed lemon juice
- 2 tablespoon of olive oil
- ¼ cup of raisins
- ¼ cup of sliced almonds
- 1/8 cup of shredded parmesan cheese

To create the dressing, add the lemon juice and olive oil in a small bowl and whisk together (no vinegar is required for this dressing). Combine the kale and apple in a large bowl. Slice and core the apples; skin can be left on or removed before adding. Add the raisins, cheese, almonds, and black pepper. Mix well, then serve.

Kale: A Versatile Superfood with Many Options
51-60. Simple Kale Recipes

Kale is one of the most nutrient-rich green leafy vegetables available. It's a hardy vegetable that can grow in harsh and cold climates, and available in several varieties, from red or red kale to light green or dark with curly leaves. All types of kale provide a wide range of antioxidants, vitamins, calcium, fiber, and protein. It's an ideal food to include in any diet, especially if you follow a plant-based way of eating. There are many uses for kale, which can be used in the following "mini" recipes:

51. Kale chips: coat one-inch leaf slices lightly in olive oil and sea salt, and roast in the oven for 8-10 minutes on 350 degrees for a light snack.

52. Use a flat kale leaf as a wrap for hummus and chili powder

53. Saute one cup of kale slices on medium heat with garlic and olive oil for a tasty side dish

54. Wrap large kale leaves around cubes of brie cheese and bake for 10 minutes

55. Saute kale with onions for a topping on a burger or sandwich.

56. Roast two large kale leaves wrapped around garlic cloves for a unique snack or side dish treat.

57. Add ¼ cup of thinly sliced kale into a cup of miso soup instead of seaweed (or with ¼ cup of dried seaweed).

58. Shred 1 cup of kale leave for a topping on soup or stir fry dishes, along with dry roasted nuts and/or dried fruits

59. Use kale leaves as a wrap for tuna or chicken salad sandwiches, instead of bread

60. Lightly roast kale leaves in a skillet, then top with 1-2 teaspoons of sesame seeds.

The following recipes focus on healthy grains and pulses, which can be easily incorporated into healthy salads as meals for any time of day. Grains tend to be filling and can satisfy hunger longer than many other foods. For this reason, grain-based recipes are ideal for long commutes or when you expect not to eat for an extended time.

61. Refreshing Quinoa Salad
- 2 cups of cooked quinoa
- 1 large cucumber, sliced into ½ or 1-inch pieces

- 1 cup of cherry tomatoes, sliced in halves
- 1 small red onion, sliced thinly
- ½ cup of dried or fresh mint leaves
- 1 teaspoon of black pepper
- 3 tablespoons of olive oil
- 2 tablespoons of dried rosemary
- 1 juiced lemon
- 1 ripe, yet firm avocado, peeled, cored and sliced into small pieces
- 3 tablespoons of red wine vinegar

To prepare the dressing, combine the vinegar, olive oil, lemon and rosemary into a small bowl. Whisk well and set aside. Cook two cups of quinoa and set aside to cool. In a large bowl, combine the quinoa, cucumbers, tomatoes, onions, mint leaves and black pepper. Mix thoroughly, then carefully sprinkle in the salad dressing, and add in the sliced avocado and serve.

62. Quinoa and Dried Fruit Salad

- 1 ½ cups of cooked quinoa
- ¼ cups of dried blueberries
- ¼ cups of dried raspberries
- 1 teaspoon of lime juice
- ¼ cups of roasted pecans
- ½ cup of crumbled feta cheese

Toss the quinoa with the dried berries in a large bowl and add in the lime juice. Top with crumbled feta cheese roasted pecans, and serve.

63. Spicy Rice Salad

- 3 cups of cooked white rice
- 1 can of black beans
- 1 cup of corn
- 1 cup of salsa
- ½ cup of shredded cheddar cheese (low sodium)
- 2 green onions, sliced
- 1 red pepper, sliced

- 1 teaspoon chili powder

Cook the rice and add to a large bowl, once it has cooled for 15-20 minutes. Mix in the black beans, corn, salsa, onions, pepper and chili powder, and mix well. Serve in bowls and top with shredded cheddar cheese. Sour cream and sliced avocado are also good options for toppings.

64. Rice, Apple and Raisin Salad

- 1 large or 2 small apples, cored and sliced
- Juice of 1 lemon
- ½ cups of raisins
- 1 cup of cooked rice
- ½ cup of freshly chopped parsley

Cook the rice and cool, then transfer to a large bowl. In a separate, small bowl, coat the apple slices in lemon juice evenly. Add the apples, raisins, and parsley to the bowl, mix and serve.

65. Roasted Almond and Rice Salad

- 2 cups of cooked rice
- 1 cup of sliced almonds (dry roasted)
- ½ cup of shredded coconut

Combine the cooked rice with shredded coconut and add ½ cup of the roasted almonds. Serve and top with the remaining dry roasted almonds.

66. Fresh Summer Salad

- 2 cups of cooked basmati rice
- 1 cup of snow peas
- ½ cup of fresh parsley, chopped
- 2 carrots, shredded
- 1 stalk of celery, sliced
- 1 small red onion, thinly sliced
- 1 red pepper, sliced
- 1 green pepper, sliced
- 1 teaspoon of black pepper

Combine the above ingredients in a large bowl and mix evenly.

Mix the following ingredients into a small bowl to make the dressing:

- ¼ cups of olive oil
- ¼ white wine vinegar
- 1 tablespoon of mayonnaise
- 2 teaspoons of honey
- 1 teaspoon of black pepper

Whisk in a small bowl, and drizzle over the salad, then serve.

67. Mediterranean Barley Salad

- 2 cups of cherry tomatoes, sliced in halves
- 1 cup of cooked barley
- ½ cups of feta cheese (crumbled)
- 1 teaspoon of black pepper
- ½ cups of black olives (pitted)
- 1 red onion, sliced
- 2 tablespoons of olive oil
- 3 tablespoons of white wine vinegar

Cook the one cup of barley in three cups of water, then remove from heat when done and cool for 15 minutes. Add the barley, feta cheese, black olives, tomatoes, and red onions into a bowl. Whisk the olive oil and wine vinegar in a small bowl and mix into the salad before serving.

68. Barley and Cucumber Salad

- 1 cup of cooked barley
- 1 large tomato, sliced
- 1 large cucumber, sliced
- ½ cup of chopped parsley
- 1 teaspoon of dried dill
- 1 teaspoon of black pepper

Combine the above ingredients and mix thoroughly. Add the following ingredients into a bowl to create the salad dressing:

- 2 tablespoons of lemon juice
- 2 tablespoons of olive oil

- 1 teaspoon of black pepper

Mix the dressing ingredients and drizzle into the barley cucumber salad, then serve.

The remaining salads combine a variety of beans, vegetables, and fruits to create unique tastes for small meals and side dishes.

69. Parsley and Bean Salad
- 2 cups of finely chopped parsley (fresh, not dried)
- ½ can of black beans
- ½ can of kidney beans
- 2 tablespoons of vinegar
- 2 tablespoons of avocado oil
- 1 tablespoon of lime juice

Combine all the above ingredients and mix well before serving.

70. Simple Cucumber Salad
- 2 medium cucumbers, sliced thinly
- ½ cup of sliced onion (yellow or white)

Combine the two ingredients in a medium bowl, and mix the following ingredients to create a dressing:

- 3 tablespoons of white vinegar
- ½ cup of dried or fresh dill
- 3 tablespoons of mayonnaise
- ½ cups of sour cream

Mix the above ingredients well, then spread evenly into the cucumber and onion blend, then serve.

71. Cucumber, Tomato, and Leek Salad
- 1 cup of cherry tomatoes, sliced in halves
- 2 medium or 1 large cucumber, diced
- 1 cup of sliced leeks (green onions can be substituted if leek is unavailable)
- 1 cup of shredded feta cheese

Combine the tomatoes, leeks, and cucumber in a large bowl, and cover with feta cheese. For additional flavor, squeeze lime juice or create a light dressing with one tablespoon of olive or avocado oil and one tablespoon of lime juice.

72. Watermelon and Cucumber Salad

- 3 cups of watermelon, cut into cubes
- 1 large cucumber, diced
- ½ cup of mint leaves
- 1 cup of crumbled feta cheese
- Juice from one lime
- 1 teaspoon of black pepper

Combine the watermelon, cucumber, mint leaves and juice from the lime in a medium bowl and mix well. Mix in the black pepper and sprinkle feta cheese over top before serving.

73. Tomato and Onion Salad

- 2 large tomatoes, sliced
- 1 small red onion, diced
- 2 teaspoons of black pepper
- 2 tablespoons of vinegar
- 2 tablespoons of olive oil

Combine all the above ingredients in a medium bowl and mix well before serving.

74. Spinach, Feta, and Apple Salad

- 1 cup of fresh spinach leaves
- 1 large crisp apple, cored, peeled and chopped
- ½ red onion, sliced
- ¼ cups of sliced almonds
- ½ cups of crumbled feta

Combine the first four ingredients in a large bowl, and mix the following to create the dressing:

- ¼ cups of olive oil
- 2 tablespoons of white wine vinegar
- 1 clove of crushed garlic
- 1 teaspoon of black pepper

- 1 teaspoon of mustard seeds

Whisk the five ingredients to create the dressing and combine it with the salad. Add the crumbled feta cheese and carefully fold in, then serve.

75. Spinach and Strawberry Salad

- 2 cups of fresh spinach leaves
- 1 cup of sliced strawberries (stems removed)
- 1 teaspoon of minced red onion
- ½ cup of dry toasted sliced almonds
- 1 teaspoon of paprika

Mix all the ingredients together, and combine the following to create the dressing:

- 1 teaspoon of pressed strawberry or orange juice
- 2 tablespoons of olive oil
- 2 tablespoons of white wine vinegar

Whisk the dressing together, and combine with the salad, then serve. Add more sliced almonds and/or strawberries as a topping, if desired.

76. Orange Spinach Salad

- 4 cups of fresh spinach leaves (baby spinach)
- ½ cup of pistachios (shelled, unsalted)
- 2 medium oranges, sliced into quarters
- 1 cup of crumbled feta cheese
- 2 pears, sliced lengthwise

Combine all ingredients, and in a separate, small bowl, prepare the following ingredients for the dressing:

- 1 teaspoon of orange zest
- 2 tablespoons of orange juice
- 4 tablespoons of avocado oil
- 1 teaspoon of honey or maple syrup

Prepare the dressing, then mix into the salad before serving.

77. Potato Salad

- 2 hard-boiled eggs
- 1 tablespoon celery seeds
- 1 teaspoon black pepper
- 1 red onion, sliced
- 2 celery stalks, sliced
- 4-5 medium potatoes, skins left on, cut into 1-inch pieces
- ½ cup of mayonnaise
- 2 tablespoons mustard
- ½ cup of sweet pickles

In a large cooking pot, bring 3-4 cups of water to a boil with the potatoes, then cover and cook for approximately 30 minutes, or until well done. Remove and drain the potatoes, set aside and cool. In a small bowl, combine the pepper, mayonnaise, mustard, celery seeds, and onion. Combine with the potatoes gently, then add the pickles. Chop the hard-boiled eggs into quarters and add into the salad, then serve immediately. This recipe can be stored in the refrigerator for up to 4 days.

78. Arugula and Alfalfa Sprouts Salad with Ginger

- 2 cups of shredded lettuce
- 1 cup of alfalfa sprouts
- 1 cup of chopped arugula leaves
- ½ cup of shredded parmesan
- ¼ cup of bacon crumbles or bacon bits

Combine the lettuce, arugula, and sprouts together and set aside. To create the dressing, whisk the following ingredients together in a small bowl:

- 1 tablespoon of honey
- ½ teaspoon of grated ginger root
- 2 tablespoons lemon or lime juice
- 1 tablespoon olive or avocado oil

Once the dressing is prepared, mix with the lettuce, arugula, and alfalfa sprouts, then toss in the bacon crumble orbits, and top with parmesan to serve.

79. Beetroot Salad with Quinoa
- 3 medium beetroots, peeled and cut into quarters
- 2 cups of spinach or arugula (or any combination of greens)
- 1 cup of crumbled goat cheese
- ½ cup of chopped walnuts
- ½ cup of cooked quinoa

In a medium cooking pot, bring 2 cups of water to boil and add the beetroots. Cook until tender, for 20-25 minutes, then remove from heat and drain. Set aside to cool for 10 minutes. Mix the greens, walnuts, goat cheese, quinoa and add the beetroot. Create a salad dressing by combining the following:

- 3 tablespoons of honey or maple syrup
- 2 tablespoons of olive oil
- 3 tablespoons of freshly squeezed orange juice
- ¼ teaspoon of orange zest

Mix the dressing with the salad, the serve.

80. Pomegranate and Arugula Salad
- Seeds of 1 pomegranate
- 3 cups of arugula leaves
- ½ cup of chopped walnuts
- 1 small red onion, sliced

Combine the pomegranate seeds with the arugula leaves and toss in the walnuts and red onion slices. To make the dressing, combine the following:

- 2 tablespoons of pomegranate juice (if there isn't enough, add orange or lemon juice)
- 2 tablespoons of honey
- 2 tablespoons of red wine vinegar

Mix the dressing and pour, blend with the salad and serve.

CHAPTER 5: RECIPES FOR POULTRY, FISH AND VEGETARIAN PROTEINS

Fish is an excellent source of calcium, protein and omega 3 and 6 fatty acids. Whether you enjoy fish on occasion or more often, it's a great food to incorporate into your diet. Just a small amount of tuna or salmon can boost your energy and provide you with a host of important ingredients. The following recipes are easy to create and require common, budget-friendly foods for the whole family.

81. Baked Salmon

This is a simple recipe prepared with butter, lemon and dill.

- 2 salmon steaks
- 2 teaspoons of softened butter
- 1 teaspoon of dill (fresh or dried)
- 1 small lemon

Preheat the oven to 350 degrees and prepare a baking pan with parchment paper, lightly coated in butter. Place both salmon steaks in the pan and sprinkle with dill. Bake for 35-45 minutes or until well done. Serve with sliced lemon.

82. Tuna Casserole

This is a hearty, filling dish that can feed a family for dinner, or serve as healthy comfort food.

- 2 cups of cooked egg noodles
- 2 cups of green peas
- 2 cans of tuna (in water, drained0
- 1 tablespoon of black pepper
- 2 cans of cream of celery soup (low or no sodium)

- ½ cup of milk
- 1 cup of almond flour
- 2 tablespoons of butter
- 1 cup of old cheddar (shredded)

Prepare a deep baking dish by lining with parchment paper and lightly coating with butter, then preheat the oven to 350 degrees. Combine the noodles, tuna, peas, celery soup, black pepper, milk, tuna, and cheddar cheese in a large bowl and mix well. Transfer the mixture into the baking dish and sprinkle almond flour over top. Bake for 20-25 minutes, or until the top is slightly golden brown, then remove, cool and serve.

83. Avocado Stuffed with Tuna

- 2 large, ripe avocados (pitted, skin removed and set aside, and flesh scooped into a small bowl)
- 1 can of tuna, drained
- ½ small onion, diced
- 1 teaspoon of olive oil
- 1 teaspoon of dill
- 1 teaspoon of chili powder
- 1 teaspoon of black pepper

In a medium bowl, combine the avocado flesh, tuna, onions, olive oil, dill, black pepper, and chili powder. Scoop into the empty avocado shells and serve. For a larger serving with more than two avocados, increase the tuna to 3 cans, and double all other ingredients.

84. Garlic Shrimp

In moderation, shrimp is a good source of healthy fats and can be a good side dish or light meal option. This dish combines the powerful flavor of garlic with butter, simmered in fresh shrimp.

- 2 cups of small shrimp, or 12-16 medium or large-sized shrimp
- ¼ cup of softened butter (unsalted)
- 2-3 cloves of garlic, crushed

Heat a skillet on medium and add the butter, then the garlic. Reduce the heat to a slightly lower setting, low-medium, and add in the garlic. Fry until tender, and garnish with dried dill and/or black pepper.

85. Coconut Shrimp

- 2 cups of large or medium uncooked shrimp
- 1 cup of shredded coconut (unsweetened)
- ½ cup of almond flour
- 2 small eggs
- 1 teaspoon of olive oil

Preheat the oven to 350 degrees and thaw shrimp, if frozen, then wash and set aside. In a small bowl, whisk the two eggs and add the olive oil. In a second bowl, combine the almond flour and shredded coconut (this will be the coating for the shrimp). Prepare a baking tray with parchment paper. Dip each shrimp into the egg and olive oil mixture, coating lightly, then coat evenly in the coconut and flour mix, and place on the tray. Repeat with all shrimp until the tray is ready. Bake for 20 minutes or until shrimp are lightly browned, then serve.

86. Mango Sauce for Shrimp

- 2 mangos, pitted, peeled and sliced
- 2 teaspoons of black pepper
- 1 teaspoon of water

Add the ingredients to a blender and pulse into smooth. Pour into a small bowl and use it as a dip for the coconut shrimp.

87. Rice Pilaf with Parsley and Dill

- 1 cup of long-grain rice
- 2 cups of water
- 1 teaspoon of dill (fresh or dried)
- 1 teaspoon of dried parsley

Bring two cups of water to boil in a small or medium cooking pot. Add the rice and reduce heat to medium heat until fully cooked.

Stir in the dried dill and parsley, then serve as aside. This dish works well with baked salmon or chicken.

88. Onion Rice Pilaf

Cook two cups of rice as directed in the above recipe. In a small skillet, fry one small sliced onion in two tablespoons of olive oil. Cook until tender, then drain any extra oil from the onions. Stir into the cooked rice and serve.

89. Fried Mushroom Rice Pilaf

Saute one cup of thinly sliced button mushrooms in a small skillet with olive oil until tender. Combine with two cups of rice and serve.

90. Coconut Rice

- 2 cups of coconut milk
- 1 cup of jasmine rice
- 2-3 tablespoons of water

Bring two cups of coconut milk and the tablespoons of water to a boil over medium heat. Pour in the rice and lower the heat, continue to stir to prevent the rice from sticking until fully cooked. Serve as a side with a meat or vegetarian entrée.

91. Chicken Fried Rice

- 2 cups of chicken broth
- 1 cup of basmati or regular rice
- 1 cup of cooked chicken (fried or baked, leftovers from a roast dinner)
- 1 teaspoon poultry seasoning
- 1 teaspoon turmeric
- Dash of black pepper
- 1 teaspoon of crushed garlic
- Half a sliced onion
- Olive oil

In a medium cooking pot, bring two cups of chicken broth to a boil, and stir in the rice. Reduce the heat and cook on medium until rice is done. Remove from heat and prepare a skillet with olive oil. Saute the garlic and onions. Cook the rice and add in the chicken, spices, and seasoning. Stir and continue to cook until all rice is coated and slightly browned. Serve in bowls and garnish with parsley.

92. Mushroom Fried Rice

Prepare the recipe by following the directions in the previous recipe. Substitute the cooked chicken for one cup of sauteed mushrooms.

93. Celery and Carrot Fried Rice

Saute sliced carrots and celery (two stalks of each) in two teaspoons of olive oil until tender, then add to the cooked rice in the skillet (follow the chicken fried rice recipe).

94. Onion Fried Rice

Following the chicken fried rice recipe, substitute one cup of fried onions (diced into small pieces).

Poultry Recipes

Chicken is an excellent source of lean protein and a versatile option for many dishes. A simple roast or stir fry can be flavored and seasoned in many ways, without high sodium or artificial ingredients.

95. Roast Chicken

Prepare a chicken by rinsing and removing the giblets. Preheat the oven to 350 degrees and combine the following ingredients in a small bowl to baste the poultry:

- 3 tablespoons olive oil
- 2 teaspoons of poultry seasoning
- ½ teaspoon black pepper
- 1 teaspoon basil

Coat the chicken in lightly with the oil mixture and place in a preheated oven at 350 degrees. Roast for 2-3 hours, checking and basting the chicken once every half hour to prevent from drying. Continue roasting until well done. Test with a fork to ensure the meat is thoroughly cooked, then slice and serve with dinner.

96. Roast Turkey

Prepare the turkey in the same way as the chicken in the recipe above, by removing the giblets and preheating the oven to 350 degrees. Coat the turkey with the following spices and ingredients:

- 4 tablespoons of olive oil
- 1 teaspoon of black pepper
- 2 teaspoons of paprika
- 1 teaspoon of basil
- 2 teaspoons of sage
- 1 teaspoon of thyme

Coat the turkey lightly before transferring to the oven. Bake for 3-4 hours, or until meat is ready and thoroughly cooked.

97. Giblet Gravy (from Chicken or Turkey)

To prepare a gravy from the giblets, add them to a skillet and heat on medium with butter. Add in the following ingredients:

- 1 cup of sliced onions
- ½ cup of sliced celery
- 1 teaspoon of thyme
- 1 teaspoon of sage
- ½ cups of sliced carrots
- 2 bay leaves
- 1 teaspoon of crushed garlic cloves (or dried garlic)
- All drippings from the turkey or chicken
- 5 cups of water

- 1 teaspoon of mustard

Reduce heat and cook for 30 minutes, then drain liquid and add the following to make the gravy:

- 3 tablespoons of gravy
- 2 tablespoons of cornstarch
- 1 teaspoon of water

Stir all ingredients in a small pot and ensure there are no lumps, then serve with roast chicken or turkey.

98. Cranberry, Orange and Pomegranate Sauce

- 2 cups of fresh or frozen cranberries
- 1 orange, freshly squeezed, including peel and pulp
- ½ cup of honey or low carb sweetener
- Seeds from ½ of a pomegranate

In a small cooking pot, combine the above ingredients and add two cups of water, or enough to cover. Cook on medium until close to boiling, then reduce to low and cook for 20-25 minutes or until all fruits are tender. Drain carefully, transfer to a jar or container and refrigerate until served with a meal.

99. Stir-Fried Chicken with Vegetables

This meal is best prepared in a large wok or skillet.

- 3 chicken breasts, boneless, cut into one-inch pieces
- 3 tablespoons of low sodium
- 1 cup of snow peas
- 1 small onion, diced
- 2 cloves of garlic, crushed
- 1 cup of bean sprouts
- ½ cup of sliced almonds
- 2 celery stalks, sliced
- 2 carrots sliced into small pieces

Heat a large wok or skillet with olive oil. Add chicken and soy sauce and cook until well done on medium. Add in the onion, garlic and cook for 5 minutes, then add the remaining ingredients and saute for 5-10 minutes until tender but crunchy. Serve over rice.

100. Stir Fry Chicken with Sliced Almonds

Prepare the recipe above and serve with dry roasted almonds.

Plant-based, Vegan Protein Recipes

Incorporating plant-based recipes into the dash diet is a beneficial way to get a lot of nutrients. Soy-based foods are full of vitamins, minerals, and protein. Tempeh and tofu are excellent meat alternatives for a vegan diet and are easy for the body to digest. If you haven't explored many plant-based options, the following soy food recipes are easy to follow and provide a good foundation for including vegan choices into your diet. As part of the Dash Diet, soy-based foods and all plant-based protein is an easier way for your body to get the nutrients needed, without the more challenging task of breaking down meat products and animal proteins. Plant foods tend to be easier to digest and keep weight manageable, which is another advantage of reducing and maintaining healthy blood pressure.

101. Basic Baked Tofu
- 1 block of a firm (or extra firm) tofu
- 1 cup of low sodium soy sauce
- 2-3 tablespoons of sesame oil

Rinse a block of tofu and slice into 2-inch cubes. Add to a resealable container. In a small bowl, combine the soy sauce and sesame oil, then pour over the tofu cubes, making sure everything is coated evenly. If needed, pour one cup of water or vegetable broth to cover. Refrigerate for a minimum of two hours or leave overnight to marinate. When ready to cook, drain the liquid, reserving just ½ cup in a bowl. Preheat the oven to 350 degrees and line a small baking dish with parchment paper. Add the tofu pieces to the pan and bake for 20-30 minutes, or until slightly browned and "crispy" or hard on the surface. The tofu should still be softer inside when sliced open. Serve the tofu as a snack, side dish or combine with other servings for lunch or dinner.

102. Sesame Baked Tofu

Following the above recipe, add a light coating of sesame seeds (approximately 1/8 cups), lightly coated in olive or sesame oil to the tofu and bake in the oven. Sesame seeds can also be dry roasted and added as a topping when serving the tofu as a dish.

103. Orange Baked Tofu

Using the basic baked tofu recipe, add 1 tablespoon of orange marmalade (unsweetened), plus 1 teaspoon of orange juice and zest:

- 1 block of tofu (extra firm tofu)
- ½ cup of soy sauce (low sodium)
- 1 tablespoon of orange marmalade
- 1 teaspoon orange juice plus zest

Coat the tofu in the above ingredients (mix in a bowl before adding) and refrigerate overnight. Bake for 25 minutes at 350 degrees.

104. Spicy Baked Tofu

Add 2 teaspoons of chili powder or paste to the basic baked tofu recipe to create a spicier version of the recipe.

105. Sweet and Sour Baked Tofu

This recipe involves more ingredients to achieve a combination of both sweet and sour, without adding sugar and preservatives. To prepare the tofu for the marinade, combine the following ingredients in a small or medium bowl:

- ½ cup of pineapple juice
- ¼ cup of rice vinegar
- 3 tablespoons low carb sweetener (or brown sugar)
- 2 teaspoons of soy sauce (low sodium)
- 1 tablespoon of tomato paste (low or no sodium)

- 1 teaspoon grated ginger
- 2 tablespoons orange juice

Whisk all the above ingredients together and cover the tofu in a resealable container. Refrigerate for two hours or overnight, then drain and serve. Reserve some of the liquid to use in the skillet to fry the tofu with vegetables and other spices if desired.

106. Sweet and Sour Skillet Tofu

Heat a skillet on medium with olive oil and add the baked tofu (sweet and sour). Reduce heat and add in the following ingredients to fry until tender, yet crispy:

- 1 small diced onion
- 1 green pepper, sliced
- 1 red pepper, sliced
- 2 cloves of garlic, crushed
- ½ cup of sliced green onions
- 2 teaspoons grated ginger

Sautee the above ingredients with the tofu, then serve with rice or as a side dish.

107. Spicy Tempeh

Tempeh is a fermented soy food, and often contains a firmer, meat-like texture than tofu. This food is high in nutrients, including B12, fiber, calcium, and protein. To prepare for marinating, mix the following ingredients in a small bowl:

- ½ cups of olive oil
- 2 tablespoons of chili paste
- 1 teaspoon of paprika
- 1 teaspoon of oregano
- 1 tablespoon of soy sauce

Combine all ingredients into a paste and baste the tempeh. Cover in a container and refrigerate for a minimum of three hours. Preheat the oven to 350 degrees and bake in a parchment paper-lined dish for 25-30 minutes.

108. Simple Baked Tempeh

- 1 cup of soy sauce (low sodium)
- 1 teaspoon of rice vinegar
- ½ cups of olive oil
- 1 teaspoon of black pepper
- ½ teaspoon of lemon juice

Combine the ingredients above into a small bowl and coat the tempeh. Refrigerate for three hours or more, then remove and bake in the oven for 30 minutes at 350 degrees. Remove and serve with a salad, as a side dish or add to a variety of other recipes.

109. Stir Fry Tempeh and Snow Peas

The simple or spicy baked tempeh will come in handy for a variety of dishes, including this easy to create a recipe that involves adding a couple of vegetables to the skillet with the tempeh.

- 2 cups of baked tempeh, cut into cubes
- 2 cups of raw snow peas
- ½ cup of sliced or slivered almonds
- Olive oil to fry
- 1 teaspoon of black pepper

Heat the skillet on medium, and add the tempeh, cooking for 10-15 minutes, then add the snow peas and black pepper, and cook for another 5 minutes or until the snow peas are slightly tender, yet remain firm and crispy. Remove from the stovetop to serve, and garnish with sliced almonds.

110-120. Simple Tempeh Recipe Ideas

The following short recipe ideas are suggestions for a variety of tempeh skillet dishes. These can also be used with baked tofu, in the same way, depending on your preference:

110. Saute 1 cup of thinly sliced button mushrooms, ¼ cup of onions with tempeh.

111. Fry 1-2 sliced green peppers to serve with tempeh or tofu, and garnish with sesame seeds.

112. Combine bean sprouts and fry lightly, then add to any combination of vegetables and other ingredients for a tofu or tempeh dish.

113. Add small broccoli and/or cauliflower florets to the skillet with a light coating of curry powder and ¼ cup of coconut milk, then add in the spicy tempeh.

114. 1 cup of spicy tempeh can be served in a bowl of ramen noodles boiled in miso or vegetable broth.

115. 1 or 2 cups of baked tempeh or tofu can be added to a bed of fresh spinach leaves, garnished with lemon or orange juice and sesame seeds or dry roasted almonds.

116. Combine spicy tempeh with one cup of coconut milk, 2 teaspoons turmeric, ¼ cup of curry paste and bamboo shoots for a unique curried dish.

117. Create a spicy fried rice dish by preserving some of the marinating liquid, and adding to one cup of cooked rice, then mixing with tempeh.

118. Add 2 teaspoons of tomato paste to the spicy or simple tempeh bake and add to pasta sauce. Serve with baked eggplant.

119. Add 1 cup of baked tofu or tempeh to a bowl of miso soup with seaweed and ½ cup of chopped green onions.

120. Serve as a filling in a wrap, with lettuce, grilled peppers and onions, and hummus.

The Plant-based Protein Power of Beans and Legumes

In addition to tofu, tempeh, and other soy-based foods, there are many options with chickpeas, beans, lentils, and other vegan options loaded with nutrients. In fact, many people can enjoy a well-balanced diet without animal products, while e experimenting with many forms of plant-based nutrients. The following dishes are simple dips, spreads, and bowls that can provide a quick boost before going to work, midway through the day or before a trip to the gym.

121. Creamy Hummus Dip

- 1 can of chickpeas, drained and rinsed
- ¾ cups of tahini softened at room temperature
- 1 tablespoon of freshly squeezed lemon juice
- 3 cloves of garlic, crushed
- 1 teaspoon of cumin powder
- 1 teaspoon of black pepper
- 1 teaspoon of sea salt
- 3 tablespoons of olive oil

In a food processor, combine the chickpeas and tahini and blend until smooth. Add in the lemon, olive oil, cumin, garlic, black pepper, and salt, then continue to blend until there are no lumps. To make this hummus dip creamier, add 1-2 teaspoons of water and blend further. Another teaspoon of tahini can also smooth the texture as well.

122. Roasted Garlic Hummus

Referring to the above recipe, prepare this hummus recipe by reducing the number of crushed garlic cloves from three to two, and roast a clove of full garlic in the oven for 15-20 minutes at 350 degrees. Remove the whole garlic and notice the cloves inside are soft and have a milder aroma. Add this to the recipe and blend with the remaining ingredients.

123. Beetroot and Red Onion Hummus

- 1 can of chickpeas
- ½ cup of tahini
- 1 cup of diced, sauteed red onion
- 1 beetroot, peeled and cut
- 1 teaspoon of sea salt

- 1 teaspoon of black pepper
- 1/8 cups of olive oil
- 1 teaspoon of cumin
- 3 garlic cloves, crushed

In a skillet or frying pan, heat oil on medium and add the red onions and beets. Cook for 10 minutes until tender, then remove from heat to cool. In a food processor, combine the chickpeas, tahini, cumin, beetroot, garlic, onions, lemon juice, and oil, and blend until smooth.

124. Pine Nuts and Hummus Dip

- ½ cups of roasted pine nuts
- 1 can of chickpeas
- ½ cup of tahini
- 3 garlic cloves, crushed
- 1 teaspoon of cumin
- 1 teaspoon of sea salt
- ½ teaspoon of chili pepper (optional)
- 2 tablespoons of lemon juice
- 3 tablespoons of olive oil

In a small frying pan, dry roast the pine nuts for 2-3 minutes, then set aside to cool. Prepare all the ingredients for the blender, adding 1/3 or ½ of the roasted pine nuts and blend until smooth. Serve and top with the remaining pine nuts. Sprinkle with sea salt or cumin.

Snacks, Dips, and Sides

125. Avocado Dip

- ½ cups of sour cream
- 2 teaspoons of thinly diced onion
- 1 ripe avocado
- ¼ teaspoon chili powder
- 1 teaspoon lime juice

Combine all ingredients in a small bowl and serve.

126. Artichoke Dip

- 2 cups of cooked spinach
- 1 can of artichoke hearts
- 2 cloves of garlic, crushed
- 1 teaspoon of parsley
- ½ cup of sour cream
- 2 teaspoons of parmesan
- 1 teaspoon of black pepper
- 1 teaspoon of thyme
- 1 cup of white beans (rinsed and drained)

Combine all ingredients in a baking dish greased with butter. Preheat the oven to 350 degrees and bake for 35 minutes.

127. Steamed Asparagus with Sliced Almonds

- 1 bunch of asparagus
- ½ cups of sliced almonds (raw or toasted)
- ½ cups of shredded parmesan

Slice one bunch of asparagus into four-inch-long pieces. Cook in a medium saucepan covered in water and steam until tender. Serve with butter and toasted almond slices. Sprinkle with parmesan cheese and serve.

128. Baked Brie Cheese

This is a simple dish to create with just one ingredient: wrap one small wheel of brie cheese in tin foil and bake for 15-20 minutes in the oven at 350 degrees. Remove, unwrap and serve as a dip.

129. Cottage Cheese and Fruit

- 2 cups of low-fat cottage cheese
- 1 cup of sliced pineapple
- 1 peeled mandarin, sliced
- ½ cups of pitted cherries

130. Broccoli and Cheese

- 4 cups of chopped broccoli florets
- 2 cups of shredded cheddar (low sodium)
- 2 teaspoons of black pepper
- 2 tablespoons of skim milk

Combine milk and cheddar in a small bowl. Steam the broccoli in a medium cooking pot until tender, then drain and transfer to a medium cooking pot and heat with butter. Add in the cheddar and milk. Stir and stew and until the cheese is melted and evenly mixed into the broccoli, then serve. Top with extra shredded cheese and pepper.

CHAPTER 6: RECIPES FOR SMOOTHIES AND REFRESHING BEVERAGES (HOT AND CHILLED)

Smoothies for all Occasions: Breakfast, Snacks and Energy Boosts

There's nothing like a rich and delicious smoothie for breakfast or as a tasty energy boost in between errands or meals. As an energy boost, smoothies are an ideal way of giving your body the fuel it needs just before the gym. If you've ever purchased a smoothie or fresh-pressed juice from a local juice bar, you would've paid more than enough for just one glass. These recipes provide a number of homemade options that will save your budget and allow you to experiment with many different flavors and ingredients.

131. Banana and Coconut Smoothie

Just one banana will provide up to one and thirty minutes of energy. Combining a banana with unsweetened coconut milk is a quick way to enjoy a boost before the gym and going for a bicycle ride.

- 1 banana
- 1 ½ cups of coconut milk
- 1-2 teaspoons low carb sweetener (optional)

Add the banana, milk, and sweetener into a blender and pulse for 30 seconds. Continue to blend, if needed, to create a smooth texture without any lumps. Add more sweetener if desired. To chill, add a couple of ice cubes, or slice the banana and freeze 2 hours before making the smoothie.

132. Mango Yogurt Smoothie

Low-fat, unsweetened yogurt is a great way to add protein, calcium, and probiotics to your smoothie. Any mango variety can be added, when they are ripe and easy to blend. This recipe includes cardamom and sweetener, both of which can be adjusted to suit your preference.

- 1 cup of yogurt (low-fat, unsweetened)
- 1 cup of almond or skim milk (unsweetened)
- 1-2 ripe mangoes (pitted, skin removed, sliced)
- 2 teaspoons of crushed cardamom pods or powder
- 2-3 teaspoons of low carb sweetener

Combine the yogurt and milk in the blender and pulse for 5 seconds, then add the ripe mangoes, sweetener, and cardamom and continue to blend for 30 seconds, then serve.

133. Peach Smoothie

If peaches are in season, they can add a wonderful flavor to a smoothie, along with a good dose of fiber. This treat can be a light dessert or enjoyed in between meals.

- 2 peaches (pitted, skins removed, sliced)
- 2 cups of almond milk (unsweetened)
- 2 teaspoons of low carb sweetener or honey

Combine the peaches and milk in the blender and pulse for 30 seconds. Add the sweetener and continue to mix for another 20-30 seconds until smooth, then serve. To chill, add two ice cubes or freeze the peach slices for two hours before.

134. Blueberry Smoothie

The sweetest berry of all, blueberries add a distinct taste to a smoothie, which doesn't require the adding of any honey, maple syrup or low carb sweeteners. The result is a fiber and antioxidant boost that works well in the morning, or at any time during the day.

- 1 cup of blueberries (fresh or frozen)

- 2 cups of almond or skim milk

Combine the berries and milk in the blender and mix until smooth.

135. Blueberry Yogurt Smoothie

To create a light breakfast and add some protein and calcium to your blueberry smoothie, thicken the recipe with a half cup of low-fat yogurt.

- 1 cup of blueberries (fresh or frozen)
- 1 ½ cups of almond or skim milk
- ½ cups of low-fat, unsweetened yogurt

Add the milk and yogurt to the blender and pulse for 15-20 seconds. Add the berries and continue to blend until smooth, then serve.

136. Blackberry, Blueberry, and Cherry Smoothie

The decadent combination of cherries, blueberries, and blackberries work together to create a sharp flavor that satisfies the taste buds and appetite. All berries can be fresh, frozen or a mix of both.

- ¾ cups of blueberries
- ¾ cups of blackberries
- ¾ cups of cherries
- 2 cups of almond or skim milk
- 1-2 tablespoons of natural or low carb sweetener

Combine all ingredients in a blender and pulse for 30-45 seconds. Continue to blend until smooth, then serve. If berries are fresh, add 2 ice cubes to chill.

137. Cherry and Banana Smoothie

Cherries are naturally sweet on their own and contain a good alkaline balance, which is good for your gut health. Adding ripe cherries to your smoothie creates a natural sweetness that eliminates the need for sugar.

- ½ cup of fresh pitted cherries
- 1 ripe banana
- 2 cups almond or skim milk

Blend all ingredients until smooth, then serve.

138. Currents and Berries Smoothie with Yogurt

Fresh currents are ideal for this smoothie, though frozen can be also used, if available.

- 1 cup of fresh or frozen black currants
- 1 cup of raspberries or blueberries (or ½ cup of both combined, fresh or frozen)
- 2 cups of almond or coconut milk
- 2 tablespoons low carb sweetener

Blend all ingredients until smooth. Add more berries or milk to thin or thicken as needed, then serve.

139. Pumpkin Spice Smoothie

- 2 cups of almond or coconut milk
- 1 cup of pumpkin puree
- 1 teaspoon of nutmeg
- 1 teaspoon of cinnamon
- ¼ teaspoon of cloves
- 3 teaspoons honey or low carb sweetener
- 1 teaspoon vanilla extract

Combine the milk and pumpkin in the blender and mix until smooth. Add the spices, sweetener and vanilla extract and continue to mix, then serve.

140. Banana and Pumpkin Smoothie

Following the above recipe, add ½ cup extra milk and 1 ripe banana, and blend until smooth.

141. Chocolate and Peanut Butter Smoothie

- 2 cups of coconut milk

- ¼ cups of cocoa powder or melted baker's chocolate
- 2 tablespoons of low carb sweetener
- 3 tablespoons of smooth, organic peanut butter (unsalted, no sugar added)
- ½ teaspoon of vanilla extract

Add all ingredients to the blender and pulse until smooth.

142. Chocolate and Banana Smoothie

Follow the above recipe, substituting the peanut butter for one banana, and adding an extra ½ cup of milk.

143. Hazelnut and Chocolate Smoothie

Following the smoothie recipe for peanut butter and chocolate, substitute the same portion with hazelnut butter and prepare.

144. Tahini and Honey Smoothie
- ½ cups of tahini butter
- ¼ cups of honey
- 2 cups of coconut milk

Blend all ingredients in a blender and serve.

145. Creamy Banana Smoothie
- 2 cups of coconut milk
- 1 ripe banana
- 2 tablespoons of sweetener

Blend all ingredients until smooth and serve.

146. Cinnamon Banana Smoothie
- 2 cups of coconut milk
- 1 ripe banana
- 2 teaspoons of cinnamon
- 2 tablespoons of sweetener

Combine into a blender and mix until smooth.

147. Pistachio Smoothie
- 1 ½ cups of almond or coconut milk

- 1 cup of crushed pistachios
- 2 teaspoons of sweetener (honey is recommended)
- 2 teaspoons of coconut or dairy cream

Blend all the above ingredients. To thicken, add more cream, then serve.

148. Banana and Pistachio Smoothie

Follow the above recipe and add one ripe banana. Blend and serve.

149. Mocha Smoothie

- ½ cup of ground coffee
- ½ cup of cocoa powder
- 2 cups of coconut milk
- 1 ripe banana
- 2 teaspoons of sweetener

Combine all ingredients into a blender and mix until smooth. Add melted chocolate instead of cocoa. To thicken, add less milk or more banana.

150. Pumpkin and Banana Smoothie

- 1 ripe banana
- 1 cup of pureed pumpkin
- 2 tablespoons of sweetener
- 1 teaspoon of nutmeg
- 1 teaspoon of cinnamon
- 2 cups of almond or coconut milk

Combine all ingredients in a blender and mix until smooth, then serve.

Fresh Pressed Juices

A glass of freshly pressed carrot and apple juice, or a refreshing drink made with mint leaves and watermelon are just samples of many delicious options for naturally prepared drinks that support the immune system.

151. Mango Carrot Juice
- One pitted mango with skin removed
- 2-3 raw carrots

In a juicer, add the two carrots and mango slices. To thin the juice, add half an apple, then serve.

152. Kale and Apple Juice
- One medium apple, cored, peeled and sliced
- 2 cups of sliced kale leaves, stems removed

Juice the kale and push into the juicer with slices of apple. Add more apple if desired, then serve.

153. Grapefruit Juice
- 2 large grapefruits

Slice two large grapefruits into quarters and squeeze or press the juice into a glass. Add ½ teaspoon of honey for a sweetener, if desired. This juice is good with the pulp included, or it can be strained and served.

154. Lemon and Apple Juice
- 3 apples, cored, peeled and sliced
- 1 lemon squeezed
- 1 teaspoon of honey

Juice all three apples, then stir the juice from one lemon and add a teaspoon of honey.

155. Ginger Carrot Juice
- One inch of fresh ginger root
- 2-3 carrots, peeled and sliced

Juice the carrots and ginger together and serve.

156. Pineapple and Coconut Juice
- 2 cups of fresh, sliced pineapple
- 1 cup of coconut water
- 1 tablespoon of coconut milk (optional)

Juice the pineapple chunks and stir in the coconut milk and

water. For a creamier drink, replace the water with coconut milk.

157. Parsley, Beet and Carrot Juice
- One small beetroot, sliced and chopped
- 2 carrots, peeled and sliced
- ¼ cup of parsley

Juice the parsley, then beets and carrots. Add some apple to sweeten the drink, if desired.

158. Turmeric, Apple and Lemon Juice
- 3 apples, cored, peeled and sliced
- Juice from one lemon
- 1 teaspoon of turmeric

Juice the apples and stir the lemon and turmeric powder. If turmeric is fresh, juice the root with apples before the lemon.

159. Watermelon and Mint Juice
- 3-4 cups of sliced watermelon
- ¼ cups of mint leaves, sliced
- ¼ cup of lemon juice

Juice all three ingredients, then serve.

160. Grape and Lime Juice
- 1-2 bunches of grapes (seeds or seedless – these will be removed in the juicer)
- ½ cup of lime juice
- 1 small apple

Juice the three ingredients, then serve.

161. Pineapple and Coconut Juice
- 2 cups of sliced pineapple
- 1 cup of coconut water or juice
- 1 teaspoon of honey
- 1 teaspoon of lime

Juice the pineapple, then add to the coconut water, honey and lime in a blender and pulse before serving. For a creamier smoothie, add coconut milk instead of juice.

162. Turmeric, Ginger and Lemon Juice

- 1 small ginger root
- 2 cups of freshly squeezed lemon juice
- 2 teaspoons of honey
- 1 small turmeric root

Juice the ginger and turmeric root and combine it with honey and lemon juice.

Natural Flavor Infused Water

Is drinking enough water each day a challenge? Most people drink less than the recommended, and often enjoy a soda, fruit juice or another flavored beverage. Getting enough water is one of the most important aspects of maintaining a balanced diet and a healthy lifestyle. If you're active and exercise regularly, a steady source of water becomes increasingly more important to avoid dehydration. A variety of natural flavors can be added to water to create a variety of tasty options. It's a better option than purchasing store-bought "flavored" water, which is often sweetened with artificial ingredients. The following infused water options are worth a try and will give your regular hydration more variety.

163. Cucumber Water

Slice one cucumber into thin disks and add to a large pitcher. Pour filtered water into the jug and chill for at least two hours to allow the cucumber flavor fuse with the water. Serve in a glass with ice.

164. Citrus Water

Add slices of orange, lime, lemon and/or grapefruit to a jug and pour water. Add some zest or squeeze a combination of citrus juice for added flavor. Refrigerate for two hours, then serve.

165. Strawberries and Cucumber Water

Add one cup of sliced strawberries and one large sliced cucumber into a pitcher and pour water into the jug. Chill for two hours, then serve with ice.

166. Lemon and Mint Water

Squeeze juice from two lemons and add 2 teaspoons of finely shredded mint into a large jug. Add two sliced lemons into the picture with the juice, mint and pour water to cover and chill.

167. Raspberry and Blueberry Water

This combination will add a naturally sweet flavor to water. Pour water over one cup of fresh raspberries and blueberries combined. Squeeze two tablespoons of orange juice, then chill and serve with ice.

168. Cantaloupe and Mint Water

Add two cups of sliced cantaloupe and a small handful of mint leaves to the bottom of a pitcher. Pour water and chill for one hour, then serve with ice and one or two leaves.

Hot Drinks

There are many hot beverages to enjoy in addition to regular tea and coffee. These varieties are excellent for the Dash diet and can be enjoyed at any time of year, including during the winter months. Most drinks offer sweetener options (either natural or low carb), though some are enjoyable without any at all.

169. Hot Mocha

This drink is easily made with freshly brewed coffee and melted chocolate or cocoa powder. There is the option to add low-fat milk or a non-dairy option:

- 2 cups of freshly brewed coffee
- 2 tablespoons cocoa powder or melted dark chocolate
- 1 teaspoon low carb sweetener (optional)
- 2 tablespoons milk

Combine the coffee with the cocoa or chocolate, sweetener and milk and use a small hand mixer to blend, then serve.

170. Hot Mocha with Cinnamon

Prepare this drink by following the recipe above and add 1 teaspoon of ground cinnamon.

171. Hot Coconut Milk Mocha

This drink is the same as above, only with the addition of ½ cup of coconut milk, warmed on the stovetop with an extra teaspoon of cocoa powder or melted chocolate.

172. Cardamom Ginger Drink

- 2 teaspoons of cardamom powder
- 2 teaspoons of ginger powder or grated ginger root
- 2 teaspoons of low carb sweetener or honey
- 2 cups of coconut or almond milk
- 1 cinnamon stick

In a small saucepan, heat the coconut milk on medium and add the spices, sweetener and cinnamon stick. Stir and cook for 15 minutes, and do not bring to a boil. When the drink is warm, remove from heat and serve.

173. Matcha Green Tea Drink

- 2-3 teaspoons of matcha green tea powder
- 2 cups of coconut or almond milk
- 2 teaspoons of low carb sweetener or honey

Add the coconut or almond milk to a small saucepan and add the matcha powder and sweetener. Cook until there is a light froth, though do not bring to a boil. Serve.

174. Apple Cider and Cranberry Drink

- Two cups of apple cider
- 1 cup of fresh cranberries
- 1 cinnamon stick

Combine the cranberries and apple cider with the cinnamon stick on medium heat on the stovetop, then serve.

175. Black Pepper and Turmeric Drink

- 2 cups of almond or coconut milk
- 2 teaspoons of turmeric
- ½ teaspoon black pepper
- 1 teaspoon low carb sweetener or honey

Heat the milk on medium, adding the sweetener, black pepper, and turmeric. Stir and continue until warm and well mixed, then serve.

Chilled Drinks

Chilled teas, coffees and a variety of other mixes that include juices, teas, and other beverages are refreshing and enjoyable. The following drinks are also healthy and provide a lot of health benefits.

176. Iced Black Tea

- 2 cups of brewed tea (with or without tea bag) with ice
- 2 teaspoons honey
- ½ freshly squeezed lemon

177. Iced Black Tea with Milk (Sweetened Tea)

- 2 cups of brewed tea with ice
- 2 teaspoons of honey or maple syrup (a low carb sweetener is also an option)
- 1/8 cups of milk (dairy or non-dairy)

178. Iced Green Tea (Sencha)

- 2 cups of steeped Sencha green tea with ice
- 2 teaspoons of honey or maple syrup
- ½ freshly squeezed lemon

179. Iced Fruit Green Tea

- 2 cups of steeped Sencha green tea with ice
- 2 teaspoons of honey or maple syrup
- 1 freshly squeezed orange
- ¼ cup of raspberries (add to the drink)

180. Iced Oolong Tea with Milk

- 2 cups of steeped oolong tea with ice
- 2 teaspoons of honey
- 1/8 cups of almond or coconut milk

181. Iced Rooibos Tea

- 2 cups of rooibos tea with ice
- 2 teaspoons of honey
- 1/8 cups of almond or coconut milk

182. Iced Coffee

- 2 cups of brewed coffee
- ½ cups of coconut milk or skim milk
- 2 teaspoons of sweetener
- 2-3 ice cubes

183. Nutmeg Iced Coffee

- 2 cups of brewed coffee
- ½ cups of coconut milk or skim milk
- 2 teaspoons of sweetener
- 1 teaspoon of nutmeg
- 2-3 ice cubes

184. Cinnamon Iced Coffee

- 2 cups of brewed coffee
- ½ cups of coconut milk or skim milk
- 2 teaspoons of sweetener
- 1 teaspoon of cinnamon
- 2-3 ice cubes

185. Iced Mocha

- 1 ½ cups of brewed coffee
- ¼ cup of melted chocolate or 3-4 tablespoons of cocoa powder
- 2 teaspoons of sweetener
- ¼ cup of skim milk, almond or coconut milk

CHAPTER 7: RECIPES FOR DESSERTS

186. Chia Pudding
- ½ cup of chia seeds
- 1 cup of coconut milk
- ½ cup of cream
- 2 tablespoons of honey or low carb sweetener
- 1 teaspoon of vanilla extract

Combine the milk and cream, then stir in the sweetener, chia seeds, and vanilla. Use a whisk to ensure all ingredients are equally mixed, then refrigerate for two hours or overnight. Serve as breakfast or a light snack or dessert.

187. Chocolate Chia Pudding
- ¼ cup cocoa powder or melted chocolate
- 1 cup of coconut milk
- ½ cup chia seeds
- ½ cup whipping cream
- 1 tablespoon of sweetener

Combine all ingredients and whisk in a medium bowl until thoroughly mixed. Chill for a minimum of two hours and serve with chocolate shavings.

188. Coconut Chia Pudding
- 1 cup of coconut milk
- ½ cup of coconut cream
- 3 tablespoons of shredded, unsweetened coconut
- 2 teaspoons sweetener
- ½ cup of chia seeds
- 1 teaspoon of vanilla extract

189. Avocado Chocolate Pudding

- 1 large avocado (ripe)
- 2-3 teaspoons of honey, maple syrup or low carb syrup
- 2 tablespoons of cocoa powder (unsweetened)

In a small bowl, mash the avocado and mix in the syrup and cocoa powder, the serve.

190. Banana-Avocado Chocolate Pudding

- 1 ripe banana
- 1 large avocado (ripe)
- 2-3 tablespoons of cocoa powder (unsweetened)
- 2 teaspoons of honey, maple syrup or low carb sweetener

Mash the banana and avocado together, or separately, then combine in a medium bowl. Add in the sweetener, cocoa powder and thoroughly mix before serving.

191. Coconut Cream Avocado Chocolate Pudding

- 2 tablespoons coconut cream (if mixed with milk or water, choose the thickest part to add)
- 1 large avocado (ripe)
- 2 tablespoons of shredded coconut
- 2-3 teaspoons of sweetener
- 2 tablespoons of cocoa powder

Mash the avocado in a small or medium bowl, then add the coconut cream, sweetener and half of the shredded coconut. Mix well, then serve with coconut shredding on top.

192. Peanut butter, Chocolate Avocado Pudding

This variation on avocado pudding adds a heaping tablespoon of peanut butter mixed with melted dark chocolate or cocoa powder, then combined with the avocado and sweetener.

- 1 tablespoon smooth, low sodium and unsweetened peanut butter
- 2 tablespoons sweetener
- 1 avocado (ripe)
- 2 tablespoons cocoa or melted dark baker's chocolate

For best results, combine the peanut butter, cocoa, and sweetener together until thoroughly blended, then in the ripe avocado.

193. Hazelnut Cocoa Banana Pudding

This variation uses the same technique to mash the avocado as the pudding base. Bananas work easily as a thickening agent for pudding and smoothies.

- 2 ripe bananas
- 1 tablespoon of hazelnut butter
- 2 teaspoons of sweetener (honey or maple syrup is recommended)
- 2 teaspoons of cocoa powder

Mix the hazelnut butter with the cocoa powder, then add the sweetener. Stir in the banana and mash until smooth. Add ½ or 1 teaspoon of coconut cream to create a slightly smoother and creamier texture.

194. Sweet Potato Pudding

A tasty, vegan treat, sweet potato pudding offers a source of fiber and vitamin A, along with a delicious flavor.

- 3 teaspoons of maple syrup
- 2 medium sweet potatoes
- 1 teaspoon of vanilla extract
- ½ cup of coconut milk
- Dash of sea salt

To prepare the sweet potatoes, preheat the oven to 400 degrees. Cover the sweet potatoes in tin foil and poke with a fork. Bake in the oven for 45-60 minutes, until soft, then remove and cool for 20 minutes. Slice the sweet potatoes and remove the flesh and transfer to the blender. Add in the coconut milk, vanilla extract and maple syrup with the sea salt and mix until smooth. Serve in a dessert bowl warm or chilled. Sprinkle nutmeg or cinnamon as a topping.

195. Pumpkin Pudding

This dessert can be served warm or chilled.

- 3 teaspoons of maple syrup or honey
- 1 can of pumpkin puree
- ¼ cup of coconut milk
- 1 teaspoon nutmeg
- 1 teaspoon cinnamon
- ¼ teaspoon cloves

Pour the pumpkin, spices, sweetener and coconut milk into a blender and mix gently. Serve in small, dessert bowls with whipped cream.

Tofu puddings are a good source of nutrients and make the process of creating a wide variety of flavors and textures easy. These recipes are prepared with soft, silken tofu, a blender, and your choice of ingredients. Berries, nuts, seeds, chocolate, nut butter, and purees can be blended in combination or on their own. The choice of sweetener is up to your own preference: add just a little honey or maple syrup, or blend with low carb sweeteners. Choose plain, unflavored tofu for best results.

196. Chocolate Tofu Pudding

- 6 tablespoons of melted baker's chocolate or cocoa powder
- 1 package of silken tofu
- 2-3 tablespoons of almond, soy or coconut milk
- ¼ cup of sweetener

Add all ingredients in a blender and mix for 1-2 minutes, until smooth. Serve in small dessert bowls.

197. Chocolate and Banana Tofu Pudding

- 6 tablespoons of melted baker's chocolate or cocoa powder
- 1 package of silken tofu
- 1 ripe banana
- 2-3 tablespoons of almond, soy or coconut milk

- ¼ cup of sweetener
- Dash of cinnamon or nutmeg

Add all ingredients in a blender and mix for 1-2 minutes, until smooth. Serve in small dessert bowls.

198. Pistachio Tofu Pudding

- 1 cup of pistachio nuts, crushed in a grinder
- 2 tablespoons of coconut milk
- 1 package of silken tofu
- 1 teaspoon of cinnamon
- 3 tablespoons of sweetener

Add all ingredients in a blender and pulse for two minutes. To ensure the nuts are well mixed, grind the pistachios into a fine paste, then mix with the remaining ingredients. Serve topped with fresh, shelled pistachios.

199. Mango Tofu Pudding

- 1 package of silken tofu
- 2 medium mangoes, peeled, sliced and pit removed
- 2 tablespoons of sweetener
- 2 tablespoons of coconut milk

Mix all ingredients into a blender until smooth and serve.

200. Mixed Berries Tofu Pudding

- 1 package of silken tofu
- 1 ½ cups of sliced strawberries, blueberries, blackberries and raspberries (or any combination of mixed berries)
- 3 tablespoons of sweetener
- 2 tablespoons of coconut milk

Combine all ingredients into a blender and mix until smooth. Serve topped with fresh berries and a dollop of coconut cream or whipped cream.

201. Hazelnut Cream Tofu Pudding

- 1 package of silken tofu

- ½ cup of hazelnut butter
- 2 tablespoons of coconut milk
- 3 tablespoons of sweetener
- ½ cups of ground hazelnuts

Combine the first four ingredients in a blender and mix. Grind the hazelnuts and add ¾ of the mix into the pudding. Continue to blend and serve with remaining hazelnuts on top of serving the dish.

202. Peanut Butter and Chocolate Tofu Pudding

- 1 package of silken tofu
- ¼ cup of smooth, unsalted peanut butter
- 1 teaspoon of sea salt
- 2 tablespoons sweetener
- ½ cups of crushed peanuts
- 2 tablespoons of almond or coconut milk
- 5-6 tablespoons of cocoa powder or melted baker's chocolate

Mix the tofu, cocoa or chocolate, sweetener and milk in a blender and pulse. Add in the crushed peanuts and continue to blend. In a separate small bowl, mix the peanut butter and sea salt. Pour the chocolate tofu pudding blend into bowls and pour, swirl the peanut butter into each serving with a fork, then serve.

203. Banana Coconut Tofu Pudding

- 1 package of silken tofu
- ¼ cup of coconut milk
- 3 teaspoons shredded coconut (unsweetened)
- 3 tablespoons of sweetener
- 1 ripe banana

Combine all ingredients in a blender, leaving 1 teaspoon of shredded coconut aside for topping. Blend until smooth, then serve in bowls and top with shredded coconut.

204. Ginger Tofu Pudding

- 1 package of silken tofu
- ½ cup of low carb sweetener or syrup
- 2 tablespoons of coconut milk or cream
- 2 teaspoons of grated ginger (fresh)

Combine all ingredients into a blender and pulse until smooth, then serve.

205. Mint Chocolate Tofu Pudding

- 1 package of silken tofu
- 3 tablespoons of cocoa powder or melted baker's chocolate
- 2 tablespoons of sweetener
- 1 teaspoon of mint extract

Blend all ingredients until smooth and serve with mint leaves and chocolate shavings.

206. Orange Chocolate Tofu Pudding

- 1 package of silken tofu
- 3 tablespoons of cocoa powder or melted baker's chocolate
- 2 tablespoons of sweetener
- 1 teaspoon of orange extract or juice
- 1 teaspoon of orange zest

Blend the ingredients together in a blender with the orange juice and zest until smooth. Serve with a topping of sliced orange or zest.

Ice Cream Recipes

Ice cream doesn't have to be an unhealthy indulgence or an expensive treat. There are two main options when considering a frozen treat recipe: dairy or non-dairy based. The type of sweetener and flavors combined can take on many forms. Sorbet is usually fruit-based with mangoes, berries and citrus fruit.

207. Raspberry Sorbet

This recipe combines two main flavors: frozen raspberries and honey or a low carb syrup of your choice. Maple syrup is also an option. To create a tasty sorbet, only a few ingredients are needed, with a blender or food processor.

- 3 cups of frozen raspberries
- 2 teaspoons lime juice
- 1 egg white
- ¼ cup of syrup or honey (a low carb syrup is a good option)

If raspberries are fresh, wash and dry them thoroughly before freezing, to avoid clumping. Store-bought berries are often best because the raspberries are frozen individually and blend well with other ingredients. In a blender or food processor, combine the raspberries with the syrup, lime, and egg white and pulse until smooth. Pour the mix into a container and freeze for 2 hours before serving. Scoop and serve in dessert cups.

208. Peach Sorbet

Peach is a naturally sweet fruit with a texture that works well with sorbet. Honey is the ideal sweetener.

- 2 peaches (ripe), pitted and sliced (frozen is preferred, though fresh peaches can be used)
- 1 teaspoon lemon juice
- 1 egg white
- 3 tablespoons of honey

Combine the peaches and lemon juice with sweetener in the blender and pulse. Add in the egg white and continue to blend. Freeze for 1 ½ hour and serve.

209. Peach and Blackberry Sorbet

The portions change slightly to incorporate a unique sweet and sour mix of peaches and blackberries in this sorbet.

- 1 peach (large, ripe), pitted and sliced

- 1 cup of frozen blackberries (fresh can also be used)
- 2 tablespoons of orange juice
- 2 tablespoons of honey or maple syrup
- 1 egg white

Add the peach and blackberries in the blender with the orange juice. Blend for 30 seconds, then add the egg white and sweetener. Continue to blend until smooth and freeze for 1 ½ hour before serving. Top with a few fresh blackberries, blueberries or a peach slice.

210. Cantaloupe Sorbet

- 4 cups of sliced cantaloupe, cut into pieces
- 1 cup of low carb sweetener or ½ cup of honey
- 1 cup of water

In a medium cooking pot, bring the four cups of water to a boil and slowly pour in the sweetener. Cook until dissolved, then remove from heat and allow to cool for 15 minutes. Pour into a blender with the chopped cantaloupe and pulse until smooth. Transfer into a container and freeze for three hours, then scoop into small bowls to serve.

211. Blueberry Sorbet

Blueberries are naturally sweet and need a little boost if anything. Orange juice and zest can add more to enhance the flavor.

- 2 cups of water
- 5 cups of frozen or fresh blueberries
- 1 cup of sweetener (low carb) or a combination of honey or syrup and sweetener (1/2 cup each)
- 2 tablespoons of orange juice
- 1 teaspoon orange zest (optional)
- 1 teaspoon lemon juice

In a small cooking pot, combine the water and sugar. Bring to a boil and stir, reducing heat and cooking until sweetener is completely dissolved. Add the lemon and orange juice and stir. Remove from heat and cool. Stir in the blueberries and orange zest.

Chill in the freezer for 2-3 hours, then serve.

212. Kiwi and Strawberry Sorbet

An excellent sweet and tangy combination, kiwi and strawberry sorbet makes a delicious summer treat.

- 2 kiwis, peeled and sliced
- 2 cups of strawberries, stems removed and sliced
- 1 ½ cups of water
- 1 cup of sweetener
- 1 teaspoon of lemon juice

Bring the water to boil on the stovetop and add the sweetener and lemon juice. Stir until dissolved and remove to cool. Add the liquid with the strawberries and kiwis to a blender or food processor and mix until smooth. If the mixture is too thin, add another kiwi or ½ cup of strawberries. Continue to blend until smooth. Freeze in a container for three hours and serve with fresh slices of strawberries and/or kiwi.

213. Watermelon Sorbet

This is a refreshing treat that serves as a summer dish or light dessert.

- 4 cups of chopped watermelon pieces
- ½ cup of low carb syrup or honey
- 2 teaspoons of lime juice
- Dash of sea salt
- ¼ cup of rum or vodka (optional)

Blend the watermelon pieces in a food processor or blender until smooth. Add the syrup, lime juice, and sea salt. If you choose to add vodka or rum, add and blend with the pureed watermelon. Freeze for 2-3 hours, then serve.

214. Rose Raspberry and Lime Sorbet

Rose flavor provides a unique twist with the raspberry and lime flavors.

- 1 cup of rose water
- 1 cup of sweetener
- 3 cups of raspberries (fresh or frozen)

Heat the water and sweetener on the stovetop until sweetener dissolves, then remove and chill. Pour the rose and raspberries into the blender and mix. Freeze for two hours, then serve.

215. Mango Sorbet

This recipe combines fresh and frozen mango, for a refreshing dessert.

- 1 cup of frozen mango slices
- 2 fresh mangoes, pitted, peeled and sliced
- ½ cup of honey or low carb sweetener
- 1 cup of ice cubes

Add all ingredients into a blender and pulse until evenly mixed. Continue to blend until smooth. If needed, add one or two teaspoons of orange or lemon juice and continue to blend.

Nut flavors make a stronger taste for ice cream, with or without dairy, and make a delicious, light dessert option.

216. Pistachio Ice Cream

This is a decadent and creamy dessert that can be enjoyed as a light dessert or a healthy, frozen treat.

- 2 cups of coconut milk
- 2 teaspoons of whipping cream or coconut cream
- 1/3 cups of sweetener (honey, maple syrup or low carb sweetener)
- 1 cup of crushed pistachios
- 1 teaspoon vanilla extract

Combine all ingredients into a blender and mix until smooth. Add to a small or medium container and freeze for two hours, then serve.

217. Hazelnut Ice Cream

- 2 cups of dairy or coconut milk
- 2 teaspoons of whipping cream
- 2 teaspoons of hazelnut butter
- 1/3 cups of sweetener
- 1 cup of crushed hazelnuts

Mix all ingredients into a blender, and blend until smooth. Add to a container and freeze for two hours. Serve with 1-2 teaspoons of crushed hazelnuts.

218. Banana and Walnut Ice Cream

- 1 ripe banana
- 2 cups of coconut milk
- ½ cup of crushed walnuts
- 2 tablespoons of sweetener

Mash the banana and add in the milk, walnuts, and sweetener. Transfer to a blender and mix until smooth. Freeze for two hours and serve.

219. Raspberry Cream Ice

- 1 cup of fresh raspberries
- 2 cups of coconut milk
- 2 teaspoons of coconut or whipping cream
- 3 tablespoons of sweetener
- 1 teaspoon of vanilla extract

Mix all ingredients in a blender and mix until smooth. Freeze for two hours and serve with fresh berries.

220. Blueberry Cream Ice

Follow the above recipe and replace one cup of raspberries with blueberries.

221. Black Current Cream Ice

Replace the berries in the above recipe with one cup of currents and increase the sweetener to ¼ cup. Blend and freeze for two hours before serving.

222. Blackberry and Cherry Ice Cream

- 1 cup of pitted cherries
- ½ cup of blackberries
- 2 cups of coconut milk
- 3 tablespoons of sweetener
- 2 tablespoons of coconut cream

Combine the above ingredients into a blender and mix until smooth. Serve after freezing for two hours.

223. Pina Colada Ice Cream

- 1 cup of chopped pineapple
- 2 cups of coconut milk
- 2 tablespoons of shredded coconut
- 1 teaspoon of orange extract
- 2 tablespoons of sweetener

Blend all ingredients until smooth and freeze for two hours. Top with additional shredded coconut when served.

224. Tahini and Maple Ice Cream

- ½ cups of tahini butter
- ½ cup of maple syrup (or ¼ cup of low carb syrup with maple flavor)
- 2 ½ cups of coconut milk
- 2 tablespoons of coconut cream
- 3 tablespoons of crushed pecans

Combine all ingredients and blend. Freeze for two hours and serve with sesame seeds.

225. Chocolate and Almond Butter Ice Cream

- 2 cups of coconut milk
- 3 tablespoons of cocoa powder or melted baker's chocolate
- 1 teaspoon of almond extract
- ¼ cups of almond butter
- 3 tablespoons of sweetener

Mix the above ingredients into a blender and pulse until smooth. Freeze for two hours, then serve.

Simple Cake Recipes

Cake recipes can be easily modified to fit into the Dash diet meal plan, including the most chocolatey and sweet varieties. Each of these recipes contains just a handful of ingredients and can be enjoyed more often than just special occasions. All the following recipes contain natural ingredients and without refined sugars or artificial flavors. Almond and/or coconut flour is substituted for whole wheat flour, to lower the carbohydrate level and increase nutrition value.

226. Vanilla Cake

If you are new to baking cake, this is a good way to begin! This recipe is an easy combination of ingredients that can be prepared and baked within an hour.

- 1 cup of low carb sweetener
- ½ cup of butter
- 2 teaspoons of vanilla or almond extract
- 2 teaspoons of baking powder
- 1 ½ cups of almond flour
- 2 eggs
- ¾ cups of coconut milk

In a large bowl, combine the sugar and butter and mash together. Preheat the oven to 350 degrees. Add the eggs to the butter and sugar mix, along with the almond or vanilla extract and continue to stir in the flour and baking powder. Grease a medium baking dish with butter and pour the mixture. Bake for 35-40 minutes, or until the top is lightly golden.

There are a few variations on the above recipe, that only require a few changes to the vanilla cake.

227. Orange Vanilla Cake

Add 2 tablespoons of orange juice and 1 teaspoon of zest to the recipe ingredients. Mix and follow the above instructions. Serve with slices of orange on top (optional).

228. Lemon Cake

Add 2 tablespoons of lemon juice and 1 teaspoon of zest or lemon extract.

229. Coconut Vanilla Cake

Measure ¼ cup of shredded coconut and add it to the recipe ingredients. When the cake is done, serve with toasted coconut flakes on top.

230. Chocolate Brownie Cake

A rich, chocolate brownie can satisfy a craving quickly, and this brownie cake is a good way to get a chocolate fix. This recipe combines just seven ingredients to create a tasty dessert or snack.

- ¼ cups of unsalted butter
- ½ cups of dark baker's chocolate
- ½ cup of low carb sweetener
- 3 eggs
- ½ cups of almond flour
- ½ cups of crushed pecans
- ¼ cups of shredded chocolate or shavings

Prepare the oven by preheating to 350 degrees. Line a baking tin with butter and set aside. In a small saucepan, melt the butter with the chocolate on low heat, to avoid burning. Stir occasionally and remove from heat when completely melted to cool. Add to a medium bowl with eggs and mix, then add the sweetener, nuts, flour, and shredded chocolate. Mix all ingredients, then pour into the baking dish. Bake for 40-45 minutes, then remove and cool slightly before slicing to serve.

There are some interesting options to explore with this simple chocolate brownie cake recipe. The next series of variations include many flavor options to add.

231. Almond Chocolate Brownie Cake

Follow the recipe above and swirl ½ cup of almond butter (softened, at room temperature) before baking for 40-45 minutes.

232. Chocolate and Peanut Butter Brownie Cake

Instead of almond butter, add the same portion, ½ cup of peanut butter and swirl into the chocolate brownie and bake for 40 minutes.

CHAPTER 8: RECIPES FOR THE SKILLET

The skillet is a great foundation to build many tasty dishes, with a variety of lean meat and vegan options. Chicken and beef are popular for stir fry meals. For plant-based diets, tempeh or tofu (see baked tofu and tempeh recipes for details) make a great option and combine well with vegetables, seeds, and nuts.

233. Basic Chicken Stir Fry

- 2 large chicken breasts, cut into one or two-inch pieces
- 2 tablespoons of soy sauce
- 1 cup of snow peas
- 1 green pepper, diced
- 1 small onion, diced
- 2 garlic cloves, crushed
- 1 cup of bean sprouts

Heat a skillet on medium with olive oil and add the chicken and soy sauce. Cook until chicken is well done, then add in the garlic and onion for another ten minutes. Continue to cook and add in the green pepper, then bean sprouts and snow peas. Cook until the vegetables are done, but slightly crunchy. Remove from heat and serve with rice or noodles.

234. Sesame Chicken Stir Fry

Follow the above recipe and replace the olive oil with sesame oil. Toss in 3 tablespoons of sesame seeds into the stir fry.

235. Sweet and Sour Chicken Stir Fry

Add the following ingredients to the above recipe:

- 1 cup of pineapple
- 2 teaspoons of honey
- 1 teaspoon of tomato paste
- 2 teaspoons of wine vinegar

236. Orange Chicken Stir Fry

Prepare the chicken by marinating in orange juice with pulp overnight. Drain the chicken from the juice and retain 2 teaspoons for the stir fry. Slice the chicken and add to the skillet with a small portion of juice to cook.

237. Basic Beef Stir Fry

- 3 cups of lean beef, sliced into small cubes
- 1 medium onion, diced
- 3 cloves of garlic, crushed
- 3 tablespoons of soy sauce
- 1 green pepper, diced
- 1 red pepper, diced
- ½ cup of sliced mushrooms

Heat a skillet on medium with olive oil and add the beef and soy sauce. Cook until well done, then add in the garlic and onions. After ten minutes, add in the remaining ingredients, with the mushrooms last. Serve with rice or noodles.

238. Spicy Beef Stir Fry

Add 2 teaspoons of chili paste and/or 1 teaspoon of chili powder to the skillet.

239. Tomato Beef Stir Fry

Add 1/8 cups of tomato paste and one fresh tomato, sliced into small cubes.

240. Portobello Mushrooms Skillet Meal

If you're looking for a departure from both meat and soy-based skillet meals, portobello mushrooms are a great alternative. They contain a meat-like texture and a pleasant flavor the combines well with many ingredients.

- 2 large or medium portobello mushrooms, sliced
- 1 green pepper, sliced lengthwise
- 1 red pepper, sliced lengthwise

- 1 yellow or orange pepper, sliced lengthwise
- 1 medium onion, diced
- 1 tablespoon of pitted, sliced black olives
- 1 teaspoon of dried parsley
- 1 small tomato, sliced
- 1 teaspoon of black pepper
- Dash of sea salt
- ½ cups of shredded mozzarella cheese

Heat a large skillet with olive oil on medium. Add the portobello mushrooms, onions and peppers together and simmer on low-medium heat. Cook for 20 minutes, then add the salt and black pepper. Lower heat and top with tomatoes, olives, and cheese. Continue to cook for another 5-6 minutes and top with parsley and additional black pepper before serving.

241. Tempeh and Eggplant Skillet Dinner

This is a simple dish that combines the fragrant flavor of eggplant with baked tempeh. Eggplant is prepared by slicing and coating with sea salt. Set aside for 20 minutes, then rinse and drain.

- 2 cups of baked tempeh
- 2 cups of sliced eggplant (already salted, rinsed and drained)
- 1 red onion, diced
- 1 red pepper, sliced lengthwise
- 2 tablespoons soy sauce
- 1 teaspoon chili seeds

Heat the skillet with sesame oil, soy sauce and toss in the tofu and eggplant. Cook until tender, then add int the onions, chili seeds, and red pepper. Continue to saute for another 15-20 minutes and serve with rice.

242. Curried Tofu Stir Fry

- 2 cups of baked tofu (basic or spicy)
- 1 ½ cups of coconut milk
- 2 tablespoons of curry powder

- 1 teaspoon of turmeric
- 1 teaspoon of chili powder
- 1 teaspoon of sea salt
- 1 teaspoon black pepper
- 1 chopped celery stalk
- 1 chopped carrot
- 1 small onion, diced
- 2 garlic cloves, crushed

Combine the tofu, curry powder, onion, chili powder, and garlic with olive oil in a skillet. Cook on medium for 5 minutes, then add coconut milk. Lower the heat and add in the remaining ingredients and cook until all vegetables are tender. Serve in bowls or with rice.

243-253. Skillet Dish Vegetable Combinations

There are many options and combinations for tasty vegetables in these "mini" recipes:

243. Carrots, celery, and basil
244. Cauliflower, curry, and turmeric
245. Potatoes, leeks and sliced green pepper
246. Sliced cabbage and curry
247. Jalapenos, okra, and red pepper
248. Spinach and okra
249. Sliced sweet potatoes and black beans with tomato paste
250. Sliced kale and red onions
251. Rosemary and potatoes
252. Parsnips, asparagus, and carrots
253. Sliced garlic, turmeric, and onions

Simple Breakfast Dishes with Eggs

254. Poached Eggs on Raw Spinach

- 2 eggs
- 1 cup of raw spinach leaves, stems removed
- ½ cup of shredded mozzarella

Bring 3-4 cups of water to a boil and gently break and add two eggs, one at a time, into the water. Cook for 10 minutes, then remove with a slotted spoon. Place over a bed of raw spinach and cover with cheese, then serve.

255. Poached Eggs and Smoked Salmon
- 2 eggs
- 3-4 slices of smoked salmon
- 1 tablespoon of capers
- 1 teaspoon dried dill
- Dash of black pepper

Prepare two poached eggs and serve over smoked salmon. Sprinkle with capers, dill, and black pepper.

256-265. Poached Eggs Breakfast Options

Poached eggs are an easy breakfast to prepare and can be served on a variety of fresh vegetables, pieces of bread or as a side to the main dish. The following poached egg dishes are "mini" recipes that can be assembled within minutes for a different combination every morning:

256. Poached eggs on rye bread

257. On a bed of alfalfa and moong bean sprouts, add two poached eggs and sprinkle with black pepper

258. Poached eggs on baked ham, sprinkled with paprika and black pepper

259. Steamed asparagus with butter, topped with two poached eggs

260. Raw or cooked kale, top with one or two poached eggs

261. Sliced tomatoes and cucumbers, with one or two poached eggs

262. Baked sweet potato (leftover from a previous meal), mashed and seasoned with oregano, black pepper, and topped with two poached eggs

263. Poached eggs with fried green peppers

264. Sauteed mushrooms and onions with poached eggs

265. Bed or rice noodles, topped with one poached egg, sprinkled

with black pepper and toasted sesame seeds

Breakfast Skillet Dishes

266. Scrambled Eggs and Spinach
- 2 eggs
- 1 cup of raw spinach
- I small onion, diced
- Dash of black pepper
- Olive oil for frying

Heat a skillet on medium heat with olive oil. In a small bowl, scramble two eggs and black pepper. Add onions to the oil and fry until tender, then add the eggs and pepper. Add in the spinach and cook on low to medium heat. Serve with toast.

267. Scrambled Eggs with Herbs
- 2 eggs
- 1 teaspoon of black pepper
- 1 teaspoon of sage
- 1 teaspoon of paprika
- 1 teaspoon of thyme
- Olive oil for frying

Whisk the eggs in a small bowl and add to a skillet heated on medium with olive oil. In a small bowl, mix the sage, paprika, thyme, and black pepper, and spoon into the scrambled eggs. Combine well and fry until done, then serve.

268. Scrambled Eggs with Dill

Just two ingredients, eggs and dill, can create a wonderfully aromatic and tasty dish. It's a simple breakfast that serves well with sliced tomatoes, cucumbers and/or avocado. Scramble two eggs with 2 tablespoons of fresh or dried dill.

269. Leftover Stir Fry and Scrambled Eggs

If there is a leftover beef stir fry or spicy chicken breast, slice, fry, and top with scrambled eggs for breakfast the next day. Skillet meals can be reheated for breakfast, as well as other meals of the day.

270-279: Scrambled Eggs Skillet Options

There are limitless options for breakfast skillet dishes, whether its leftover stir-fried vegetables or fresh herbs and spices. The following "mini" recipes can provide a few options:

270. Cubed ham and scrambled eggs
271. Fresh basil and eggs
272. Fried green peppers with scrambled eggs
273. Turmeric and curry with scrambled eggs
274. Egg whites scrambled with sliced kale
275. Refried black beans, salsa, and scrambled eggs
276. Scrambled eggs tossed with 1 teaspoon of ranch dressing, cucumbers and sliced tomatoes for a breakfast bowl
277. Scrambled eggs mixed with tomato paste and basil
278. Sliced jalapeno peppers with scrambled eggs
279. Scrambled eggs topped with sliced avocado and sesame seeds.

CHAPTER 9: RECIPES FOR SPECIAL OCCASIONS

280. Rice Pudding

- 2 cups of rice
- 2 cups of coconut milk
- 1 tablespoon of butter
- 1 teaspoon salt
- ½ cups of raisins
- 1 egg
- 1 teaspoon vanilla extract
- ½ cup of low carb sweetener
- 2 teaspoons of cinnamon

In a small saucepan, combine the milk, rice, and butter and cook until tender. Reduce heat and add in the egg, vanilla extract, and sweetener. Continue to cook on low-medium until all ingredients are fully cooked and mixed. Remove from the heat and chill, then mix in the raisins and top with cinnamon before serving.

281. Rice Pudding with Mango

Prepare the rice pudding in the above recipe and omit the raisins. Transfer the cooked rice pudding into a pan and layer with fresh mango slices on top. Sprinkle with sesame seeds.

282. Rice Pudding with Pistachios

Follow the basic rice pudding recipe and add one cup of pistachios instead of raisins.

283. Rice Pudding with Sliced Almonds

Prepare from the basic rice pudding and add one teaspoon of almond extract and top with roasted sliced almonds.

284. Eggnog Recipe

- 3 cups of milk (skim or coconut milk)

- 1 cup of heavy cream or coconut cream
- 4 egg whites
- 4 egg yolks
- 1/3 cups of sweetener
- 3 ounces of bourbon or rum

Combine all but the last two ingredients into a blender and mix until smooth. Slowly add in the sweetener, then eggs, until completely blended. Gradually add the bourbon or rum, then serve.

285. Cranberry Chutney

- 1 cup of water
- ¾ cups of sweetener (raw sugar or honey)
- 1 apple, cored, peeled and chopped
- 3 cups of fresh cranberries
- ½ cups of vinegar
- 1 teaspoon of cinnamon
- ½ teaspoons of ginger
- ¼ teaspoons of cloves
- ½ teaspoons of allspice

Bring the water to a boil and add the sweetener to a medium saucepan. Simmer until sweetener is dissolved. Add the remaining ingredients and continue to simmer until softened. Cool at room temperature and serve, or chill in the refrigerator.

286. Mint Chutney

- 1 ½ cups of mint leaves
- 1 bunch of cilantro leaves
- 1 teaspoon of sea salt
- 1 small onion, diced
- 1 teaspoon orange juice
- 1 tablespoon tamarind juice
- 1/3 cups of water

Combine all ingredients into a food processor and blend until smooth.

287. Roasted Peaches and Pears

- 2 peaches, pitted, peeled and sliced
- 2 pears, sliced in half
- 2 teaspoons of honey
- 1 teaspoon olive oil

Prepare a small baking tray and add parchment paper. Preheat the oven to 350 degrees. Lightly coat the paper with olive oil and place the pears and peaches on the tray. Bake for 15-20 minutes or until tender.

288. Baked Apple with Cinnamon
- 5-6 apples, cored, peeled and sliced
- 2-3 tablespoons cinnamon
- 2 tablespoons brown sugar or low carb sweetener
- 2 teaspoons of olive oil

Line a small baking tray with parchment paper and lightly grease with olive oil. Preheat the oven to 350 degrees. Thinly slice the apples and layer the dish. In a small bowl, mix the sweetener and cinnamon and coat the top layer. Bake for 30-35 minutes until apples are tender and topping is crispy.

CHAPTER 10: BONUS RECIPE IDEAS

(approx. 30-40 recipes and variations)

289. Kale Chips

Kale is an excellent and easy vegetable to create chips with and make a tasty replacement for high sodium potato chips as a snack. They are portable and can be enjoyed on the go or at home to satisfy a craving. Kale chips contain all the calcium, antioxidants and fiber baked as when they're fresh.

- 1 bunch of kale, stems removed and sliced into one or two-inch pieces
- ¼ cup of avocado oil or olive oil
- 1 tablespoon extra fine sea salt or pink Himalayan salt

Wash and slice the kale leaves. Ensure they are dried before lightly coating in olive oil and sprinkling with salt. Place the prepared kale on a large baking sheet lined with parchment paper and baked in a preheated oven for 8-10 minutes at 350 degrees. Check closely between eight and ten minutes, to ensure kale chips are not burnt. Serve as a light snack.

290. Parmesan Kale Chips

- 1 bunch of kale, stems removed and sliced into two-inch pieces
- ¼ cup of avocado oil or olive oil
- 2 tablespoons dried parmesan cheese
- Dash of sea salt

Prepare the kale leaves and ensure they are dry before coating lightly with oil. In a small bowl, combine the parmesan cheese and sea salt. Mix well, then sprinkle over each of the leaves. Bake on a parchment paper-lined baking tray for 8-10 minutes, or slightly longer, if needed. Ensure the chips are dried and crispy without burning. If they are wet, the baking time cook exceeds

10-12 minutes.

291. Cumin Kale Chips

- 1 bunch of kale, stems removed and sliced into two-inch pieces
- ¼ cup of olive oil
- 1 teaspoon cumin
- ½ teaspoon chili pepper (optional)

Prepare the kale leaves and combine the cumin powder and chili pepper in a small bowl. If using cumin seeds, crush them before mixing. Lightly coat each kale leaf with olive oil, then sprinkle with the cumin and chili pepper mix. Bake for 8-10 minutes. Ensure that the cumin seeds are dry and crushed before coating. Replace the ½ teaspoon of chili pepper with garam masala or sea salt, if desired.

292. Curry Kale Chips

Curry powder is an easy way to add a strong, sharp spice to the soup, stir fry and stews, and kale chips can be added to the list. This variation of the basic kale recipe replaces sea salt with curry powder. If desired, combine a dash of sea salt or pink Himalayan salt with 1 ½ teaspoon of curry powder, then coat the kale before baking. Cooking time is approximately 8-10 minutes.

293. Garam Masala Kale Chips

For a twist on kale chips, coat in 1-2 teaspoons of garam masala with olive oil and bake for 8-10 minutes. Combine curry powder, sea salt and garam masala for a unique blend.

294. Turmeric and Chili Pepper Kale Chips

Turmeric is a strong antioxidant, with a mild flavor that can be used as a flavoring with sea salt or spiced with chili pepper. Coat the kale chips and bake for 8-10 minutes.

295. Roasted Chickpeas

If you want a small burst of protein-energy in the form of a snack, roasted chickpeas are a great option.

- 1 can of chickpeas, drained and rinsed
- 2 tablespoons olive oil
- 2 teaspoons of sea salt
- 2 teaspoons of black pepper

Preheat oven to 350 degrees. Pour rinsed and drained chickpeas into a large bowl. In a small bowl, combine the olive oil, black pepper and sea salt. Mix well, then pour and evenly coat the chickpeas. Prepare a baking tray with parchment paper and place all chickpeas on the tray. Bake for 30-35 minutes, or until lightly crispy and toasted. Remove from the oven and cool before serving. Refrigerate or store in an airtight container and enjoy for up to one week.

296. Spicy Chickpeas

Add some heat to the crispy chickpeas with cayenne pepper or chili powder.

297. Curried Cabbage

- 3 cups of finely shredded cabbage (green or savoy cabbage)
- 2 tablespoons of olive oil
- 2 teaspoons of turmeric
- 2 teaspoons of curry powder
- 1 teaspoon chili powder

Heat a skillet on medium with olive oil. Add the cabbage to the pan and saute for 5 minutes. In a small bowl, mix the spices together and pour into the skillet, evenly coating the cabbage while continuing to cook for another 10 minutes. Remove from heat and serve as a side dish.

298. Cabbage in Tomato Sauce

- 2 cups of shredded cabbage
- 1 large tomato, diced

- 1 small onion, diced
- Olive oil for frying
- 2 teaspoons of black pepper
- 1 cup of pureed tomatoes (unsalted0
- 1 teaspoon dried basil
- 1 teaspoon dried oregano

Prepare of the skillet on medium heat and add olive oil, then the shredded cabbage. Cook for five minutes, then add in the spices, followed by the diced tomatoes and puree. Reduce the heat and continue to cook for 15-20 minutes.

299. Cabbage in Tomato Sauce and Lean Ground Beef

Prepare the above recipe and combine it with cooked lean ground beef.

300. Roasted Eggplant

- 1 eggplant, sliced in half
- 2 teaspoons sea salt
- ½ cup of tomato sauce (unsalted)
- 2 teaspoons olive oil

Preheat the oven to 350 degrees. Slice the eggplant in half and coat the inner flesh with salt and set aside. After 20 minutes, rinse and drain. Place both halve on a baking tray lined with parchment paper and bake for 40-45 minutes. In the meantime, warm the tomato sauce on the stovetop. Remove the eggplant from the oven and serve with the sauce poured over. Sprinkle with cheese and serve.

301. Roasted Kale and Garlic

- 5-6 cloves of garlic
- 1 bunch of kale (curly)
- 1/8 cups of olive oil

Coat the inside of a baking pan with olive oil and divide the kale leaves. Remove the kale stems and place them into the pan, along with the garlic cloves. Preheat the oven to 350 degrees. Bake for 20-25 minutes and serve as aside.

302. Stuffed peppers
- 4 large green peppers, sliced in half with seeds removed
- 1 pound of cooked ground beef (lean or extra lean)
- 1 cup of cooked rice
- 1 small diced onion
- 2 garlic cloves, crushed
- 1 teaspoon black pepper
- 3 tablespoons tomato paste

In a medium bowl, combine the beef, rice, onion, garlic, black pepper and tomato paste. Mix well and stuff each half of pepper. Preheat the oven to 350 degrees and bake for 30 minutes and serve.

303.-307. Loaded Baked Potato Recipes

With just one baked potato, there are many options for toppings. To prepare, wash and peel 4-5 potatoes, or leave the skins on. Bake in an oven for 60 minutes at 350 degrees. Potatoes generally take 45-65 minutes to bake, depending on the size. Smaller potatoes may be done within 45 minutes. Remove from the oven and remove the tin foil. Allow to cool for 10 minutes, then slice in half to add fillings or toppings:

303. Sour cream (low-fat), green onions and black pepper
304. Steamed broccoli, shredded cheddar cheese, and butter
305. Baked or stir-fried cauliflower with brie cheese
306. Cheddar cheese with bacon bits or crumble
307. Ranch dressing with fried onions

308. Avocado Toast on Rye
- 2 slices of rye bread
- 1 avocado, pit removed and sliced (firm, but ripe)
- 2 teaspoons of butter
- 1 teaspoon of black pepper

Toast both slices of rye bread, butter and layer with ripe avocado slices. Top with black pepper.

309. Spicy Avocado Toast on Rye

Follow the above recipe and top with black pepper and cayenne pepper.

Trail Mix Recipes

Trail Mix is an excellent snack that goes a long way to satisfy the appetite and your body's nutrition needs within just a few handfuls. These snacks are excellent for hiking, walking, commuting or long cycling trips. A good trail mix will include nuts, seeds, dried fruits, and various other flavors, such as cocoa or chocolate chips, shredded coconut, and fruit chips. The amount of variety is limitless, and each trail mix recipe can be a new creation, differing from the previous one. The following recipes provide many options and combinations to explore, all of which support the health and dietary goals of the Dash diet.

310. Chocolate and Peanut Trail Mix
- 1 cup of unsalted peanuts (raw or dry roasted)
- ½ cups of chocolate chips
- ½ cup of walnuts or pecans
- ¼ cups of prunes or dates, sliced

311. Coconut and Pineapple Trail Mix
- 1 cup dried pineapple cubes
- ¼ cups of apple chips
- 1 cup of dried coconut chips
- ½ cups of sliced or slivered almonds

312. Pistachio Trail Mix
- 1 cup of pistachio nuts (shelled, raw and unsalted)
- ½ cups of hazelnuts
- ½ cups of yogurt-covered raisins
- ¼ cups of cocoa or chocolate chips

313. Pre-Workout Trail Mix
- ½ cup of crushed macadamia nuts
- ½ cup of chocolate-covered peanuts
- ½ cups of coconut chips
- ¼ cup of banana chips

- 2 teaspoons raisins

314. Spicy Trail Mix
    - 1 cup of unsalted peanuts
    - 1 teaspoon chili powder
    - ½ cup of shelled pistachios
    - 1 cup roasted almonds

Sandwich Recipe Ideas

Sandwiches can be enjoyed in many forms such as wraps, flat-bread, submarines or open-faced. Choosing a nutritious bread is important, with whole grains and seeds. Ingredients should be whole and unrefined as much as possible. Rye, flaxseed, spelled and whole wheat are all good options. If you need to limit carbohydrates, wheat or gluten, there are many gluten-free and low carb options emerging in natural food markets and grocery stores. The following sandwich recipes are excellent for lunch and light meals or can be enjoyed as dinner during a busy day.

315-3. Sandwich Recipes and Ideas

315. Rye bread with smoked salmon, a light spread of mustard and capers

316. Sourdough bread with sliced cheddar and tomatoes.

317. Toasted whole-grain toast with sliced avocado and tuna salad

318. Tuna salad wrap with sliced lettuce, diced onions and green peppers and dash of chili pepper

319. Rye bread with low-fat cream cheese, sliced cucumber, and black pepper

320. Whole wheat wrap with hummus and roasted red peppers

321. Toasted whole grain bread with goat cheese and cranberry chutney

322. Wrap with gouda cheese, roasted pear, and a dash of sea salt

323. Toasted rye bread with butter, fresh basil leaves, and tomato slices

324. Submarine (whole wheat) filled with baked turkey slices,

mozzarella cheese, spinach leaves, and avocado.

325. Wrap with fried onions, roasted eggplant, hummus, and chili pepper

326. Toasted rye with oven-baked brie cheese and arugula

327. Wrap with brie cheese, roasted pear, alfalfa sprouts, and fresh blueberries.

328. Flatbread with beetroot hummus and kale chips

329. Hot sandwich on flatbread: turkey breast with giblet gravy and black pepper

330. Tuna salad with arugula on sourdough bread

331. Pine nut hummus on rye with black pepper

Granola Recipes

For breakfast, snacks or a meal replacement, granola is a quick way to fill up on energy fast for a jog or cycling. It's a good way to get a lot of nutrients and can be modified to include many or minimal ingredients. The following recipes offer many ideas for flavor pairings and taste to explore.

332. Basic Granola Recipe
   - 2 cups of whole oats
   - 2 egg whites
   - 2 teaspoons of honey
   - ½ cups of raisins
   - ¼ cups of sliced almonds
   - 2 teaspoons of cinnamon

Whisk the two egg whites in a small bowl, then add the honey. Add all other items in a large bowl and mix well. Drizzle the honey and egg white mixture and coat evenly. Preheat the oven to 350 degrees and prepare a baking tray by lining with parchment paper. Cover the tray in the mixture and bake for 25-35 minutes, until lightly toasted. Remove, cool and serve with yogurt, on its own as a snack or in a bowl with milk.

333. Cocoa Granola Recipe
   - 2 cups of whole oats

- 2 egg whites
- 2 teaspoons of honey or maple syrup
- ½ cups of chocolate chips
- 2 teaspoons of cocoa powder

Whisk the two egg whites in a small bowl and add in the honey or maple syrup. In a large bowl, combine the oats, chocolate chips, and cocoa powder. Drizzle the syrup or honey and egg white mixture and coat evenly. Preheat the oven to 350 degrees and prepare a baking tray by lining with parchment paper. Cover the tray in the mixture and bake for 25-35 minutes, until lightly toasted. Remove and cool before serving.

334. Coconut Granola

- 2 cups of whole oats
- 2 egg whites
- 2 teaspoons of maple syrup
- ½ cups of shredded coconut (unsweetened)

This is a simple version of the recipe that combines shredded coconut with oats and maple syrup. Mix the ingredients together with the egg whites and bake for 30 minutes until toasted.

335. Mixed Berry Granola

- 3 cups of whole oats
- ½ cups of dried cherries
- ¼ cups of dried blueberries
- ¼ cups of dried raspberries
- 1 cup of banana chips
- 2 teaspoons finely shredded coconut
- 2 teaspoons of honey
- 3 teaspoons of butter

Combine the whole oats, dried fruits and banana chips with the shredded coconut. In a small bowl, combine the honey and butter and mix well. Blend both bowls until evenly coated. Bake the granola on a tray for 35 minutes or until toasted. Serve with yogurt or as a cold cereal or snack.

336. Chia Seed Granola
- 1 cup of whole oats
- 1 cup of thinly sliced almonds
- ½ cups of chia seeds
- 2 teaspoons of cinnamon
- 2 teaspoons of honey
- 2 egg whites

Combine the oats and almonds into a medium bowl with the chia seeds. Mix the egg whites and honey in a separate bowl and blend with the oats and chia. Bake for 25-35 minutes until toasted.

337-347.: Granola Recipe Combinations

There are many other granola combinations to explore with oats, chia seeds, and other ingredients. For less whole wheat and gluten, replace oats with more chia seeds, almonds, cashews, and other nuts.

337. Oats dried ginger and honey
338. Chia seeds, slivered almonds, hazelnuts, and maple syrup
339. Oats, chocolate chips, shredded coconut
340. Sliced almonds, chia seeds, cashews, pistachios, and honey
341. Oats, hemp seeds and maple syrup
342. Chia seeds, honey and hemp hearts
343. Chia seeds, turmeric, dried coconut slices, and banana chips
344. Oats, sesame seeds, chia seeds, honey
345. Hazelnuts, cocoa powder, chocolate chips, and oats
346. Oats, dried pineapple slices, dried mango slices, and honey
347. Sliced almonds, cinnamon, and nutmeg

CHAPTER 11: 22-DAY DASH DIET MEAL PLAN

Starting a Dash Diet Meal Plan

Beginning a meal plan is easier than you may think, especially when there are many recipes as food options to choose from. The following daily meal plans are a guide to beginning a new, healthier way of eating.

Days 1 to 7 of the Dash Diet Plan

Day	1. Monday	2. Tuesday	3. Wednesday	4. Thursday	5. Friday	6. Saturday	7. Sunday
Breakfast	Scrambled eggs with spinach	Chia seed pudding (any flavor)	Fresh yogurt and fresh fruit	Poached eggs and rye bread	Avocado on toast	Banana and chocolate smoothie	Poached eggs with smoked salmon
Lunch	Tuna salad	Toasted rye with brie and cranberry chutney	Miso soup with ramen noodles	Kale salad with blueberries	Spinach salad	A toasted submarine with lettuce, tomato, avocado, and chicken breast	Tempeh skillet dish
Snack	Trail Mix	Apple	Kale chips	Orange	Tomato soup (broth with ½ cup of low sodium tomato juice)	Roast chicken with mint chutney	Curried cabbage on the stovetop with roasted chickpeas
Dinner	Roast chicken dinner	Egg drop soup with leftover roast chicken	Beef and barley stew	Baked tofu with coleslaw	Butternut squash soup	Tuna casserole	Ginger carrot soup
Dessert	Raspberry sorbet	Peach sorbet	Vanilla cake	Chocolate tofu pudding	Peach smoothie	Pistachio smoothie	Chocolate brownie cake

Days 8 to 14 of the Dash Diet Plan

Day	8. Monday	9. Tuesday	10. Wednesday	11. Thursday	12. Friday	13. Saturday	14. Sunday
Breakfast	Chia seed pudding (any flavor)	Mocha smoothie with boiled eggs	Scrambled eggs with turmeric, with sliced tomatoes	Avocado on toast with basil leaves	Granola and yogurt	Poached eggs with spinach and rye bread	Pumpkin smoothie
Lunch	Spicy cucumber and tuna salad	Miso soup and baked salmon	Garlic shrimp with arugula salad	Curried tempeh with snow peas	Spinach salad with roasted almonds	Kale salad with crumbled feta and pomegranate seeds	Stir-fried beef with vegetables
Snack	Kale chips	Apple	Kale chips	Pomegranate	Roasted chickpeas	The cup of yogurt with blueberries	Fresh peach
Dinner	Chicken broth with egg drop	Kidney bean stew	Rice, raisin and apple salad with miso soup	Broccoli and cheese bake	Kale parmesan chips	Roast kale and garlic	Roast turkey dinner with sides
Dessert	Rice pudding with mango	Blueberry sorbet	Walnut and Banana Ice Cream	Chocolate mint tofu pudding	Yogurt and mango smoothie	Baked apple and cinnamon	Chocolate hazelnut pudding

Days 15 to 21 of the Dash Diet Plan

Day	15. Monday	16. Tuesday	17. Wednesday	18. Thursday	19. Friday	20. Saturday	21. Sunday
Breakfast	Poached eggs with salmon, kale and rye bread	Granola and fresh raspberries with yogurt	Avocado stuffed with tuna	Chocolate chia seed pudding	Scrambled eggs with spinach	Yogurt and peaches and mixed berries	Boiled eggs with black olives and cucumber
Lunch	Stir-fried chicken with rice	Chicken fried rice and vegetables	Coconut shrimp with ginger carrot soup	Beef broth with vegetables	Spicy rice salad	Chili with sour-dough toast	
Snack	Pomegranate	Chili and cumin kale chips	Coleslaw and dried fruits	Sliced avocado	Trail mix (any flavors)	A cup of yogurt with blueberries	Sweet potato pudding
Dinner	Roast chicken dinner with quinoa salad	Potato and leek soup	Tuna and cucumber salad	Chili pepper miso soup	Sauteed portobello mushrooms	Tempeh and eggplant skillet dinner	Baked salmon with onion rice pilaf
Dessert	Roasted pear and peaches	Tahini and maple smoothie	Peanut butter and chocolate smoothie	Pina colada ice cream	Rice pudding with cinnamon	Cherry and ba-nana smoothie	Mocha with nutmeg and coconut milk

Dash Diet Meal Plan: Day 22

Day	22. Monday
Breakfast	Eggs in a skillet with leftover stir-fried vegetables
Lunch	Spinach salad with crumbled feta and fruit
Snack	Sliced pineapple
Dinner	Egg drop soup
Dessert	Pumpkin chia seed pudding with nutmeg

Designing your own custom meals and ideas

Creating your own meals and custom combinations can be a lot more interesting when you have a lot of options to work with, and only use a few items in combination. To make the best out of a new plan, consider simply cooking or preparing two or three items together, and it this way, you can create your own ideas for a new type of dish or taste that may be unique in itself, while still providing the best health options available, such as the following:

348-357. Two or Three-Item Recipe Ideas for the Frying Pan or the Skillet:

348.Carrots and sesame seeds

349.Snow peas and slivered almonds

350.Chicken breast and pineapple

351. Watercress and soy sauce

352.Stewing beef with tomato sauce and chili pepper

353. Baked chicken breast sautéed with pineapple slices

354. Spinach with brie cheese

355. Sliced garlic gloves with celery

356. Fresh portobello mushrooms with fresh parsley

357. Caramelized onions with green peppers

There are often good last-minute solutions that can make a great snack or idea when combining many ingredients together, as long as you have a solid, nutritional base, such as yogurt or milk, to build a smoothie or a slice of bread or grain. Sometimes the items leftover in a refrigerator can create more than you realize, such as balanced snacks or light meals. For example, one cup of plain yogurt can go a long way with a few fruits and/or vegetables:

358. 1 cup of sliced cucumbers over one or two cups of plain yogurt

359. Sliced almonds and crumbled ginger cookies over yogurt, as a snack

360. 2 teaspoons of orange juice and maple syrup sprinkled over two cups of plain yogurt

361. Mint leaves and sliced oranges topped over yogurt or vanilla ice cream

362. Chocolate chips in a cup of yogurt with honey or maple syrup

363. Leftover granola and banana chips mixed with yogurt

364. Sliced mandarins with yogurt

Cream cheese is another great base for building snacks and light meals from, including salads, fruit plates and as a side dish. You may want to add the following dishes together as a snack, or as a quick cream-cheese cake filling. For each of these recipes, blend together the ingredients:

365-373. Cream cheesecake and dip "mini" recipes

365. Blend one cup of cream cheese with ½ cup of raspberries (fresh or frozen)

366. Mix sliced fresh dill with cream cheese for a dip

367. Steamed asparagus and black pepper with cream cheese

368. Blend one cup of cream cheese with blueberries (fresh or frozen)

369. Wrap cream cheese into smoked salmon wraps

370. Sliced pickles with cream cheese

371. Blend one cup of pumpkin puree with two teaspoons of allspice and one cup of cream cheese

372. Mix together one cup of cream cheese with melted chocolate or two tablespoons of cocoa powder

373. Spread cream cheese on slices of cucumbers and garnish with parsley or dill

374-386. Cheesecake cups as a "mini" dessert

Plain cream cheese definitely has its advantages, especially considering the different flavoring options you can choose. In its plain state, it's also an accommodating food, as it can be purchased as a low-fat item or as a vegan, plant-based version. All types of this product can be fused together to create these small, tasty and filling cheesecakes, which are formed into small muffin cups and frozen or refrigerated for ease. The following list of ingredients is for a variety of flavor options to try with your next package of cream cheese.

374. Orange juice, honey, and lemon juice (plus zest from one lemon and orange)

375. Melted chocolate and chocolate chips

376. Fresh strawberries (stems removed) sliced, plus one tea-

spoon of maple syrup

377.   Coconut milk (one teaspoon), the juice from one lime and 2 tablespoons of shredded coconut.

378.   Almond butter, cocoa powder, and honey

379.   Blueberries (fresh or frozen), honey and vanilla extract

380.   Pistachios and honey

381.   Crushed hazelnuts and honey

382.   Maple syrup and cinnamon

383.   Lime and lemon juice, plus zest and honey or low carb sweetener

384.   Crushed peanuts and cocoa powder, plus honey

385.   Mint extract and cocoa powder with low carb sweetener

386.   Orange extract and cocoa powder with honey

Fat Bombs are popular recipes for the ketogenic or low carb diets, which offer a minimal amount of ingredients combined into small, bite-sized treats for the refrigerator or freezer. These treats are tasty, and often use low carb sweeteners or a small amount of natural sugar, such as agave, honey or maple syrup. They are fat "based", meaning one key ingredient is a healthy fat which pumps the nutrient value and supports a diet where sugar and carbohydrates are very low.

The following recipes are either mixed in a blender or a small bowl and frozen in a small ice cube or silicone tray containers for the freezer. They must be frozen before consuming, as they contain a lot of natural fats, and don't remain solid for long at room temperature. They are a good option during the summer months as well.

387-400: Fat Bomb Recipes for Low Carb Diets

387.   Coconut oil, coconut cream and shredded coconut (Coconut fat bombs)

388.   Cocoa powder, coconut cream, and coconut oil (Chocolate-coconut fat bombs)

389.   Hazelnuts, coconut cream and coconut oil (Hazelnut fat bombs)

390.	Frozen blackberries, blueberries, cherries, with coconut oil and cream (mixed berries fat bombs)
391.	Lime juice, zest, cream cheese, and coconut oil with low carb sweetener
392.	Lemon juice, zest, cream cheese and coconut oil with low carb sweetener
393.	Peanuts with cocoa powder, coconut, oil, and low carb sweetener
394.	Pistachios, cardamom, coconut oil, and cream
395.	Honey, coconut oil and cream
396.	Maple syrup, coconut oil, cream
397.	Pumpkin puree, nutmeg, cinnamon, and coconut oil and cream
398.	Cinnamon, coconut oil and cream
399.	Nutmeg, coconut oil, and cream
400.	Cocoa powder, coconut oil, and cream

401-___: Simple Two-Item Recipe Items for on the Go

If you only have a few minutes to get ready and need to put together a quick snack or light meal, consider these options. Sometimes, it may seem impossible to decide which items are a good fit, especially when there are a variety of food items that are seemingly random and may not seem like they work together. You may be surprised how well these items work!

401.	Goat cheese, cranberry chutney wrapped in lettuce
402.	Basil leaves and cheddar cheese
403.	Sesame seed sprouts with peanuts
404.	Feta cheese with black olives
405.	Sliced kale with cherries
406.	Roasted chickpeas and mozzarella cheese
407.	Sliced carrots and gouda cheese
408.	Almonds and blueberries (dried or fresh)
409.	Walnuts and prunes
410.	Pecans and banana chips
411.	Dried coconut slices and dried cherries

412.   Dried cranberries and mint leaves
413.   Sliced cucumbers and parmesan cheese slices
414.   Sesame seeds with chocolate chips
415.   Rice pudding with dried fruits (combine leftovers)
416.   Chia pudding with sliced mangoes
417.   Fresh pear with leftover coconut rice
418.   Crushed peanuts with rice pudding
419.   Granola and yogurt with chia seeds
420.   Cottage cheese with fresh pineapples
421.   Mint leaves and cucumbers
422.   Sliced peaches and pears
423.   Leftover stewed apples and cinnamon with cheese
424.   Banana chips and dark chocolate
425.   Dried mango with raisins
426.   Feta cheese with fresh cherries
427.   Fresh dill with hummus wrapped in flatbread
428.   Roasted eggplant in a lettuce wrap
429.   Curried cabbage with raisins and chickpeas
430.   Baked spicy tofu (leftover) with mint chutney

If you're looking for quick trail mix options to give you a quick source of energy for the next workout, these are easy and don't require any cooking time or baking. Simply combine and mix for the go.

431-437: Simple Trail Mix Recipes made in Five Minutes for On the Go

431.   Macadamia nuts with yogurt covered peanuts
432.   Black licorice, raisins, and dark chocolate
433.   Almonds, yogurt covered raisins, and chocolate chips
434.   Dried mangoes, prunes and walnuts
435.   Apple chips, low sodium pretzels, and parmesan shreddings
436.   Kale chips, almonds, raisins
437.   Slivered almonds, pistachios and pumpkin seeds

438-453.: Chia Seed Pudding Toppings and Alternatives

Chia seed pudding is featured as one of the most healthy light meal, breakfast and dessert options. Chia seeds are full of calcium, protein, and fiber. Just a small serving of this nutrient-dense dish can provide a lot of benefits and fill up quickly, which means there will likely be plenty of leftovers to work with and add toppings to. Consider a plain, vanilla variety of chia pudding for toppings, or combine a variety of trail mix or dried fruit and nut options for chocolate chia and other flavored chia puddings.

438.   Crushed pistachios and maple syrup on vanilla chia pudding
439.   Peanuts topped on chocolate chia seed pudding
440.   Roasted pumpkin seeds on chia seed vanilla pudding
441.   Hemp hearts on chocolate chia seed pudding
442.   Flax seeds and cinnamon on vanilla chia seed pudding
443.   Shredded coconut on berry or vanilla chia seed pudding
444.   Toasted almond slices and raisins on chia pudding
445.   Carob chips on chocolate chia pudding
446.   Coconut chips on chocolate chia pudding
447.   Bacon bits and caramel pieces on vanilla chia seed pudding
448.   Green tea matcha powder on vanilla or berry chia pudding
449.   Fresh raspberries on any flavor of chia pudding
450.   Honey coated oats on chia pudding
451.   Sliced apples and lemon juice on vanilla chia pudding
452.   Toasted almond slices and cinnamon on chia seed pudding
453.   Sliced strawberries on berry or vanilla chia pudding

454-__: Simple Sandwich Ideas

Creating simple sandwiches can be easier than the traditional ingredients while using up some leftovers and enhancing a typical meal into something tasty and fun to enjoy. Once you become familiar with and use a number of different Dash diet recipes, you'll re-invent the way sandwiches are assembled, including wraps, crepes, and flatbread.

454.   Coconut cream blended with blueberries (spread on

crepes)

455.   Cream cheese topped with prunes and maple syrup

456.   Hummus topped with parsley and chili pepper

457.   Leftover roast chicken or turkey with cranberry chutney and sliced cheddar

458.   Cheddar with sliced roast beef and mint chutney

459.   Roasted pear mixed with cream cheese on rye

460.   Fresh raspberries mixed with cream cheese and mint leaves

461.   Turkey or pork bacon, well-cooked, crumbled and combined with cranberry chutney and cream cheese.

462.   Peanut butter with cocoa powder and honey

463.   Hazelnut butter with melted chocolate and maple syrup

464.   Tahini butter mixed with maple syrup on rye

465.   Cream cheese topped with sliced green onions

466.   Canned sardines on rye with sliced onions and chili peppers

467.   Ripe avocado spread topped with bacon bits

468.   Hummus spread topped with grilled vegetables

469.   Artichoke dip and black pepper

470.   Cream cheese topped with cucumbers and cherry tomatoes, sliced in half

471.   Roasted eggplant and sprouts

472.   Spicy hummus spread and sliced jalapeno peppers

473.   Sliced cucumbers and shredded goat cheese

474.   Sliced pickles (low sodium) on top of artichoke dip mixed with cream cheese

475.   Tuna salad with sliced onions and dill, ½ teaspoon lemon juice

476.   Roast chicken (leftover) poured over flatbread and covered in giblet gravy

476.   Egg salad with chili pepper and parsley

477.   Boiled eggs sliced and topped on rye with sliced tomatoes and pepper

478.   Roasted sweet potato mixed with plain hummus on a wrap

479.   Crumbled feta cheese with sweet potato on rye

When you're finished for the day and need to unwind, a cup of hot tea with herbs is the best way. These simple steeped tea options are excellent for good health and supporting your immune system. Teas can be prepared with a tea bag or in a dried form, steeped for a minimum of five minutes, then strained and flavored

480.-503: Herbal and Flavored Teas

480.   Hibiscus tea and lemon
481.   Oolong tea and honey
482.   Rooibos tea with maple syrup and almond milk
483.   Black tea with skim milk and honey
484.   Green tea with honey
485.   Rosehip tea with mint and honey
486.   Lemon and honey in hot water
487.   Mint tea with honey
488.   Ginger tea with honey
489.   Ginger and green tea with honey
490.   Black tea, milk, and cocoa powder
491.   Green tea, milk, and honey
492.   Turmeric, ginger, and honey
493.   Green and mint tea
494.   Camomile tea with honey (or plain)
495.   Rosewater with chamomile tea
496.   Aloe juice mixed with green tea
497.   Ginger tea with aloe juice
498.   Black tea with grated ginger
499.   Jasmine tea with maple syrup
500.   Jasmine green tea with honey
501.   Masala chai tea with milk and honey
502.   Turmeric and masala chai tea with coconut milk and honey

Alcoholic Beverages

On occasion, enjoying an alcoholic beverage can be a healthy part of the Dash diet. The key is to avoid sugar and artificial flavors, by using only pure forms of liquor, without sugar, and adding a simple juice or milk base

503-520: Mixed Drinks for the Dash Diet

503.   Rum with coconut milk and vanilla extract
504.   Mango juice with vodka
505.   Masala chai with coconut milk, cardamom, and rum
506.   Dry, red or white wine
507.   Coconut and pineapple smoothie with rum
508.   Watermelon juice with vodka
509.   Lime juice with rum
510.   Lemon and lime mixed with vodka
511.   Raspberries in scotch
512.   Sliced oranges in vodka
513.   Turmeric milk tea with rum and low carb sweetener
514.   Blueberries in scotch
515.   Almond milk and cocoa powder with cinnamon and rum
516.   Mango and yogurt smoothie with rum
517.   Banana, coconut and mango smoothie with vodka
518.   Coconut milk with pistachios and rum
519.   Carrot and mango juice with vodka
520.   Ginger carrot juice with rum

Frequently Asked Questions

The Dash Diet is a well-known and researched diet that has helped many people achieve a better way of living and eating to curb and prevent further medication conditions while helping them to thrive and enjoy a healthy way of eating. Choosing nutritious options may be more commonplace to some people, while others may struggle with deciding what to eat and how to build their daily and weekly meal plans. Recipes create a good start, though it takes time to fully become accustomed to eating and living differently than before, especially if this change is major and involves a complete overhaul of a previous diet! The following questions and answers will provide further guidance and planning assistance to building and following a healthy diet customized for your lifestyle while adhering to the Dash Diet guidelines.

Question: Does the Dash Diet allow for the accommodation of allergies, or food sensitivities?

Answer: Yes. For every recipe or meal option, there is an ingredient that can be replaced with a gluten-free item, for examples, such as oats (there are gluten-free options available), or replacing a slice of bread with a wheat-free or low carb wrap. Throughout this book, both natural and low carb sweeteners are provided as alternatives to sugar, to reduce and avoid refined ingredients. This is especially important for regulating insulin levels and maintaining a healthy blood sugar level.

Question: Is this diet safe for people who have type 2 diabetes?

Answer: It's a safe diet, and in fact, it is recommended for the prevention and treatment of type 2 diabetes, as it aims to control sugar intake and insulin levels, without too much variance. Sources of sugar should be limited, and as natural as possible, from fruits and natural syrups, as opposed to refined and packaged sugars. The recipes in this book also include mostly natural, whole foods that can be easily located and purchased in the produce and fresh food sections of any grocery store, which makes the Dash diet easy to shop for.

Question: Is the Dash diet safe for children under 18 years old?

Answer: It's not necessary for children to follow this diet unless it is recommended by a doctor or medical professional, and because it doesn't require strict calorie reduction or similar restrictions, it is relatively safe for anyone to use.

Question: Is the Dash diet considered a long-term way of eating or just temporary?

Answer: It's a "lifestyle" diet and more than just a short-term fix! Eating healthy should be one of the top priorities in living a healthy life, and this is no exception. When you focus on making dietary changes for the long term, you tend to take them more seriously and will want to work towards improvements on a continual basis. For example, some of the recipes in this diet can easily replace what you may currently choose for meals, making them a more nutrient-rich option, over time, you may experiment with new ideas and ingredients to gradually make improvements over time and customize towards your own tastes.

Question: Are there any drawbacks to following the Dash diet?

Answer: As with any diet, some recipes may not be suitable for some people with specific health conditions or may conflict with certain medications. For this reason, it is advised to consult with a doctor prior to beginning or trying any new diet.

Question: Is it necessary to become vegan to reach the full potential of the Dash diet, or can this level be achieved while including meat in the diet?

Answer: It is not required to follow a strict vegan or plant-based diet under this plan, though there are many benefits to this way of eating. Plant-based foods are easier on the digestive system and are better absorbed and processed by our bodies. This makes it easier to get the most out of the nutrients in our food. If you choose to keep meat within your diet, there are plenty of options in the Dash diet, as long as lean meats are chosen and reduced in portion size. Balance is the key idea when it comes to which foods we include, whether they are animal or plant-based sources of nutrients.

Question: Is it safe to drink alcohol in moderation or only on rare occasions?

Answer: In small amounts, alcohol can be enjoyed as a part of an occasional indulgence. Avoid drinking sugary liqueurs and choose clear drinks with your own choice of juice, or simply enjoy as is. One of the best options is dry wine, which can be red or white wine, enjoyed with a meal.

Question: Should all salt be avoided, or is it permissible to enjoy a small amount every day?

Answer: Our body needs sodium as part of a healthy diet, though unfortunately, many packaged foods are saturated in sodium. As long as most (if not all) of your foods are fresh and without artificial flavors, the dangers of consuming too much sodium are much lower and your heart health and blood pressure should remain within a healthy level. Moderation is best, and using small amounts (teaspoon or less) for one meal will ensure you get just the right amount. Most natural foods we eat contain enough sodium on their own. Once you become accustomed to eating a low sodium diet, it will become easier to enjoy foods with their own flavor!

Question: How much sugar is too much and when should it be avoided?

Answer: Avoid all refined and processed sugars, which are going to cause a spike in blood glucose and impact insulin levels. Many natural fruits, such as oranges, berries, pineapples, and watermelon are sweet and can be added to recipes without the help of a sweetener. Low carb sweeteners are another good option, as they do not impact blood sugar levels and provide an alternative to sugar without the adverse effects of artificial sweeteners. Honey and maple syrup are good sources of natural sweeteners and contain some nutritional benefits as well. Regardless of which sweetener you choose, keep the dose low and minimal.

Question: How many eggs can be consumed daily?

Answer: Eggs are nutritious, and as long as they are part of a high nutrient diet with fiber, they can be safely enjoyed every day. For best results, limit the eggs to 2-3 within one day, and change your breakfast options often, switching eggs for cereal, fresh fruit, yogurt and chia pudding. Boiled eggs are an excellent snack on the go, and pair well with fruits and vegetables. While eggs can be enjoyed each day, it's best not to exceed eating two or three at once.

Question: Are there any herbs or spices that should be avoided on the Dash diet?

Answer: Some types of chili pepper and certain spices may have the effect of raising blood pressure in some people. Unless you have a specific health condition that can be adversely impacted by a specific herb or supplement, most of them are safe and beneficial for your health. If in doubt, research different sources and check with your doctor, just to be certain.

Question: What is the difference between dark and milk chocolate? Does it matter which one I use in recipes?

Answer: Dark chocolate is lower in carbohydrates, sugars, and additives than milk chocolate. For this reason, it's often the best choice. Cocoa powder is available unsweetened and included in many recipes in this book. Baker's dark chocolate is another good option. It can be melted in milk and sweetened with honey or maple syrup.

Question: Is there enough protein in nuts and seeds for a vegan diet? Should I also include soy food options?

Answer: If you are interested in following a plant-based diet, consider all of your options and try as many vegan foods as possible. Soy foods such as tofu and tempeh are excellent sources of protein, however, nuts and seeds can provide a wealth of other nutrients in a similar way (calcium, protein, mineral, vitamins, and fiber) which makes them a good substitute for meat. Chia seeds, for example, are considered a superfood for this reason. Just a small amount can provide a good portion of your daily nutrients. If you are not allergic to soy, it's worthwhile to try various forms of tofu, tempeh and miso, and different recipes. Overall, the best way to make the most out of a vegan diet is by trying new foods and getting used to many flavors, textures, and options.

Question: Should portion control be a factor for more than just lean meats? Should I be limiting the amount of each food item and recipes I try and is there a guideline to follow?

Answer: Generally, as long as you are incorporating a lot of natural foods in your diet, there is little danger of overeating. If you have (or had) a habit of overeating, stick with just one plate per sitting or meal, to avoid overindulging. If you're eating whole foods that are full of nutrients, you will naturally feel fuller faster, because the foods are not processed and it takes longer for your body to process and digest. On the other hand, fast foods and meals with high fructose corn syrup and other artificial ingredients can cause you to eat more because these types of foods do not make you feel satisfied sooner. This can result in eating more when you're already physically full, even if this is not the sensation.

Question: How do I avoid choosing the wrong foods when traveling or visiting another region or country where my regular meal options are not available?

Answer: If in doubt, choose the freshest food possible. If you travel to an area where the climate is colder and there are fewer options for fresh foods, select options with the least amount of sugar and processed ingredients. Choose wholegrain bread, fish, frozen vegetables and fruits as much as possible. It's also important to adapt and accept that sometimes choosing a food outside of your eating plan may be required, and this is only temporary. When it comes to vacation, it's best to enjoy yourself and return to your way of eating when you return from the trip. For many destinations, there are a growing number of options available, from vegan to gluten-free and low carb. You'll likely find a suitable variety in most places, as more people are becoming aware of the importance of diet and accommodating for different ways of eating. If in doubt, choose plant-based bean dishes and grains.

These will fill you quickly and satisfy your appetite longer.

Question: Are there limitations for older adults and the types of foods they can choose in the Dash diet?

Answer: Unless a specific medication has an interaction with a specific food, or unless you have an allergy and/or a condition that requires avoiding certain meals, there should be no limitations due to age. The Dash diet is a good way of eating for all age groups and doesn't hinder any growth or development process in children or young adults. It's important to choose the most nutrient-rich foods in the diet, in order to get the most out of your food options.

Question: Is the Dash diet affordable?

Answer: Yes, the Dash diet can be easily made into a budget-friendly grocery experience, whether its for individuals, couples or a family. Anyone can easily adapt to the various foods and options within the diet because there are actually more items to choose from than you may realize. Many ingredients can be purchased in bulk and in small amounts if you want to try them first. Since you'll be choosing more foods outside of the package, you'll have more freedom to control how much or little you buy according to your own taste.

Question: Is it important to be active and exercise with the Dash diet?

Answer: Exercise is an important part of a healthy lifestyle, whether its low impact, moderate movement or high impact. Keeping active is one way to stay fit and regular your metabolism. The Dash diet will support an active lifestyle because it provides all the nutrients needed to build muscle, tissue and a strong body and mind.

Question: How successful is the Dash diet?

Answer: The Dash diet is successful for anyone who wants it to work for them! If you are committed to getting and staying healthy, following the diet is just one way of doing this. You'll want to focus on key reasons why the diet is a great choice for anyone, to help you follow your goals:

- Fresh and natural foods are the most important. Build your diet around whole foods.
- Focus on the taste and enjoyment of food, instead of rushing to eat. If you are in a hurry, keep your meal light and easy to digest.
- Don't worry about dietary myths and scare tactics about eating too much or little. This diet lets you focus on keeping it natural, simple and tasty
- Choose what's right for you, and try new options and meals as often as you can. The more you enjoy eating well, the more benefits you will discover in life and health.